GETTING RESEARCH FINDINGS
INTO PRACTICE

GETTING RESEARCH FINDINGS INTO PRACTICE

Edited by Andrew Haines and Anna Donald

BMJ
Books

© BMJ Publishing Group 1998
BMJ Books is an imprint of the BMJ Publishing Group

First published in 1998
by BMJ Books, BMA House, Tavistock Square,
London WC1H 9JR

British Library Cataloguing in Publication Data

A catalogue record for this book is available from the
British Library

ISBN 0-7279-1257-7

Typeset, printed and bound in Great Britain by
Latimer Trend & Company Ltd, Plymouth

Contents

Contributors

David Armstrong, Reader in Medical Sociology, Department of General Practice, United Medical and Dental Schools of Guy's and St Thomas', London, UK

Ione Auston, Librarian, National Information Center on Health Services Research and Health Care Technology (NICHSR), National Library of Medicine, Washington DC, USA

Lisa Bero, Associate Professor, Institute for Health Policy Studies and Department of Clinical Pharmacy, University of California, San Francisco, USA

David Braunholtz, Senior Research Fellow, Department of Public Health and Epidemiology, University of Birmingham, Birmingham, UK

Jiri Chard, Research and Development Project Officer, Department of Public Health and Epidemiology, University of Birmingham, Birmingham, UK

Neil Craig, Lecturer in Health Economics, Department of Public Health, University of Glasgow, Glasgow, UK

Tony Dans, Associate Professor, Clinical Epidemiology Unit and Section of Cardiology, College of Medicine, University of the Philippines, Manila, Philippines

Rumona Dickson, Lecturer in Research Synthesis, International Health Division, Liverpool School of Tropical Medicine, Liverpool, UK

Anna Donald, Clinical Lecturer, Department of Epidemiology and Public Health, University College London Medical School, UK

Vikki Entwistle, Research Fellow, NHS Centre for Reviews and Dissemination, University of York, York, UK

Paul Garner, Senior Lecturer in International Health, International Health Division, Liverpool School of Tropical Medicine, Liverpool, UK

Julie Glanville, Information Service Manager, NHS Centre for Reviews and Dissemination, University of York, UK

J A Muir Gray, Director of Research and Development, NHS Executive, Anglia and Oxford Old Road, Oxford OX3 7LF

Roberto Grilli, Head, Unit of Clinical Policy Analysis, Laboratory of Clinical Epidemiology, Instituto di Richerche Farmacologiche "Mario Negri", Milan, Italy

Jeremy Grimshaw, Programme Director, Health Services Research Unit, University of Aberdeen, Aberdeen, UK

Gordon Guyatt, Professor of Medicine, Departments of Medicine and Clinical Epidemiology and Biostatistics, McMaster University, Hamilton, Ontario, Canada

Andrew Haines, Professor of Primary Health Care, Department of Primary Care and Population Sciences, Royal Free and University College London Schools of Medicine, UK

Margaret Haines, Principal Adviser to the Library and Information Commission (formerly the NHS Library Adviser), London, UK

Emma Harvey, Research Fellow, Department of Health Sciences and Clinical Evaluation, University of York, York, UK

Brian Haynes, Professor of Clinical Epidemiology and Medicine, McMaster University Faculty of Health Sciences, Hamilton, Ontario, Canada

Ellen Hodnett, Professor and Heather M Reisman Chair in Perinatal Nursing Research, University of Toronto, Toronto, Ontario, Canada

Rajendra Kale, Consultant neurologist, Inlaks and Budhrani Hospital Pune, India

R J Lilford, Director of Research and Development, NHS Executive, West Midlands Region, Department of Health; Professor of Health Services Research, University of Birmingham, Birmingham, UK

Theresa M Marteau, Professor of Health Psychology, Psychology and Genetics Research Group, United Medical and Dental Schools of Guy's and St Thomas', London, UK

Ruairidh Milne, Visiting Senior Lecturer in Public Health Medicine, Wessex Institute for Health Research and Development, Winchester, Southampton, UK

Sandy Oliver, Research Fellow, Social Science Research Unit, London University Institute of Education, London, UK

Andy Oxman, Director, Health Services Research Unit, National Institute of Public Health, Oslo, Norway

S G Pauker, Professor and Vice Chair, Department of Medicine, New England Medical Center, Tufts University, Boston, Massachusetts, USA

D L Sackett, Professor of Medicine and Director, Centre for Evidence based Medicine, University of Oxford Nuffield Department of Medicine, John Radcliffe Hospital, Oxford, UK

Rodrigo Salinas, Neurologist and Manager of the District Effectiveness Project, Department of Neurological Sciences, University of Chile, Santiago, Chile

Trevor A Sheldon, Professor and Director, NHS Centre for Reviews and Dissemination, Wentworth College, University of York, York, UK

Vivienne van Someren, Consultant Paediatrician and Senior Lecturer in Child Health, Department of Child Health, Royal Free Hospital and School of Medicine, London, UK

Amanda Sowden, Senior Research Fellow, NHS Centre for Reviews and Dissemination, University of York, York, UK

S E Straus, Deputy Director of Clinical Medicine, Centre for Evidence-based Medicine, University of Oxford Nuffield Department of Medicine, John Radcliffe Hospital, Oxford, UK

Matthew Sutton, Research Fellow, National Primary Care Research and Development Centre, University of York, York, UK

Paul Taylor, Lecturer. Centre for Health Informatics and Multiprofessional Education, University College, London, UK

CONTRIBUTORS

Mary Ann Thomson, Senior Research Fellow, Health Services Research Unit, University of Aberdeen, Aberdeen, UK and Assistant Clinical Professor, School of Rehabilitation Science, McMaster University, Hamilton, Ontario, Canada

Jeremy Wyatt, Fellow in Health and Public Policy; Director, Health Knowledge Management Programme, School of Public Policy, University College, London, UK

1 Introduction

ANDREW HAINES AND ANNA DONALD

Interest in how to promote the uptake of research findings has been fuelled by a number of factors. There are, for instance, well-documented disparities between clinical practice and research evidence of effective interventions. Examples include management of cardiac failure and secondary prevention of coronary heart disease, atrial fibrillation, menorrhagia, and a number of interventions in the area of pregnancy and childbirth.[1-4] Additionally, there has been a growing awareness of the need to demonstrate that public money spent on research and development results in benefits for patients. In the UK, the advent of the National Health Service (NHS) Research & Development Programme has led to greater involvement of NHS personnel in setting priorities[5] and the establishment of a programme to evaluate different methods of promoting implementation of research findings.[6] There has also been work to develop the concept of payback on research[7] which has resulted in a framework to assess the benefits arising from research.

At the same time, it has become clear that reliance on the passive diffusion of information to keep health professionals up to date is doomed to failure in a global environment in which around two million articles on medical issues are published annually.[8] There is also growing awareness that conventional continuing education activities, such as conferences and courses which focus largely on the transfer of knowledge, have little impact on the behaviour of health professionals.[9] The circulation of guidelines without an implementation strategy is also unlikely to result in change in practice.[10]

Health professionals need to plan for a rapid rate of change in knowledge which is likely to persist throughout our professional lifetimes and which encompasses not only diagnostic techniques, drug therapy, behavioural interventions, and surgical procedures but also ways of delivering and organising health services and developing health policy. Many health professionals already feel overburdened and undersupported and therefore a radical change in approach is required so that health professionals can manage change rather than feeling like its victims. A number of steps are necessary in order to support this process.

1

1. Keeping abreast of new knowledge

Health professionals need valid and relevant information available at the point of decision making without appreciable delay. Currently, despite extensive investment in information technology, this is not widely available. Relatively simple prompting and reminder systems can improve clinicians' performance[11] and prices of useful databases such as "Best Evidence" (which comprises *Evidence based Medicine* and the *American College of Physicians Journal Club* on CD-ROM) and the Cochrane Library are little more than those for journal subscriptions. There are an increasing number of journals such as *Evidence based Medicine* which summarise important papers in a rigorous fashion and present the results in a way which busy clinicians can rapidly digest. The NHS Reviews and Dissemination Centre in York compiles a range of systematic reviews relevant to clinicians and policy makers. Nevertheless, many clinicians still do not have access to such information[12] and more needs to be done to provide a wider range of high quality information which is useable in practice settings.

Librarians' roles are rapidly changing, for example in North America some are involved in clinical practice through programmes such as "literature attached to the chart" (LATCH).[13] In such programmes, hospital librarians participate in ward rounds and actively support clinical decision making at the bedside. Requests for information are documented in the notes in the articles that are subsequently delivered to the ward. Such programmes could be introduced elsewhere with appropriate evaluation, but information support is also needed for primary care which is currently woefully undersupported. Moreover, in the UK many health professionals such as nurses may not be permitted to enter their hospital library as they are not formally affiliated with the medical body that funds them.

2. Implementing knowledge

Research findings can influence decisions at many levels – individual patient care, practice guidelines, commissioning of health care, prevention and health promotion, policy development, education, and clinical audit – but only if we know how to translate knowledge into action. The acquisition of database searching and critical appraisal skills should give health professionals greater confidence in tracking down and assessing quality of publications, but this does not necessarily help the application of new knowledge to day-to-day problems.[14] Much attention has been given to the use of "Best Evidence" during the consultation with individual patients using the approach of evidence based medicine derived largely from epidemiological methods.[15,16] However, many decisions in clinical medicine also require organisational change for their implementation. Even a step as simple as ensuring that all patients with a past history of myocardial infarction are offered aspirin requires a number of steps to be taken, including identification of the patient, making contact with them, explaining the rationale, checking for contraindications, and prescribing the drug or asking the patient to purchase it over the counter. Furthermore, health professionals have their own experiences, beliefs, and perceptions about appropriate practice and attempts to change practice which ignore these factors are likely to founder. This awareness has led to greater emphasis on the understanding of social, behavioural, and organisational factors which may act as barriers to change.[17] Improved understanding requires insight from a number of fields, including education, psychology, sociology, anthropology, information technology, economics, and management studies.

A wide spectrum of approaches and interventions for promoting implementation has been used which is underpinned by a number of theoretical perspectives on behaviour change, such as cognitive theories which focus on rational information seeking and decision making; management theories which emphasise organisational conditions needed to improve care; learning theories which lead to behavioural approaches involving, for example, audit and feedback; and reminder systems and social influence theories which focus on understanding and using the social environment to promote and reinforce change.[18]

Clearly, these approaches are not mutually exclusive. For example, the transmission of information derived from research to single practitioners or small groups of health professionals (educational outreach or academic detailing) clearly has a strong educational component but may also include aspects of social influence interventions[19] by, for example, pointing out the use of a particular treatment by local colleagues. The marketing approach used by the pharmaceutical industry to promote its own products depends on segmentation of the target audience into groups that are likely to share characteristics that can be used to tailor the message.[20] Such techniques might be adapted for non-commercial use within the NHS. The evidence for the comparative effectiveness of different approaches and interventions is still patchy and will be reviewed in Chapter 4. It seems likely that in many cases a combination will be more effective than a single intervention.[21] It follows from the above that no single theoretical perspective has been adequately validated to guide the choice of implementation strategies.

The study of the diffusion of innovations, by which new ideas are transmitted through social networks, has been influential in illustrating those who adopt new ideas early tend to differ in a number of ways from later adopters, for example having more extensive social and professional networks.[22] However, much of the innovations literature has a "pro-innovation" bias with the underlying assumption that innovations are bound to be beneficial. In health care the challenge is to promote the uptake of innovations that have been shown to be effective, to delay the spread of those that have not yet been shown to be effective, and to prevent the uptake of ineffective innovations.[23]

Although a range of actors can promote the uptake of research findings, including policy makers, commissioning authorities, educators, and provider managers, it is by and large clinicians and their patients who implement findings. Having demonstrated a gap between current and desired practice a number of steps need to be taken in order to get research findings into practice (Box 1.1). A number of characteristics of the "message" also need to be considered (Box 1.2) and may influence the degree to which it is taken up in practice.

Box 1.1   Steps to promoting the uptake of research findings

- Define the appropriate "message", i.e. information to be used.
- Decide which processes need to be altered.
- Involve the key players, i.e. those who will implement change or who are in a position to influence the changes.
- Identify the barriers to change and how to overcome them.
- Decide on specific interventions to promote change, e.g. guidelines, educational programmes, etc.
- Identify levers for change, i.e. existing mechanisms which can be used to promote change (for example financial incentives to attend educational programmes, placing of appropriate questions in professional examinations).
- Determine whether practice has changed along the desired lines – the use of clinical audit to monitor change.

The choice of key players will be dependent upon the processes to be changed, for example in primary care nurses and practice administrative staff should in many cases be involved in addition to the general practitioners since their cooperation will be essential for effective organisational change. If the innovation involves the acquisition of specific skills, such as training in procedures, then those who organise postgraduate and continuing education are also key players.

Definition of barriers to change and the development of strategies to overcome them are likely to be of key importance in promoting the uptake of research findings. Some examples of barriers to the application of research findings to patients are given in Box 1.3. Chapter 10 proposes a conceptual framework for analysing and overcoming barriers. Since some of the strongest resistance may be related to the experiences and beliefs of health professionals, the early involvement of key players is essential in

---

Box 1.2   Important characteristics of the "message"

Aspects of content

- Validity
- Generalisability (i.e. settings in which it is relevant)
- Applicability (i.e. patients to whom it is relevant)
- Scope
- Format and presentation (e.g. written or computerised guidelines, absolute versus relative risk reductions)

Other characteristics

- Source of the message (e.g. professional body, Department of Health)
- The channels of communication (i.e. how it is to be disseminated)
- The target audiences (i.e. the recipients)
- Timing of initial launch and frequency of updating
- The mechanism for updating the message

---

trying to identify and, where appropriate, overcome such impediments to change.

Interventions to promote change must be tailored to the problem, the audience, and the resources available, for example educational outreach may be particularly appropriate for updating primary care practitioners in the management of specific conditions because they tend to work alone or in small groups. Guidelines based on research evidence may be developed and endorsed by national professional organisations and adapted for local use as part of clinical audit and educational programmes. Barriers need to be reviewed during the process of implementation as their nature may change as the process develops.

3. Linking research with practice

There needs to be closer links between research and practice so that research is relevant to practitioners' needs and practitioners are willing to participate in research. While there is evidence that researchers can be "product champions" of their work,[24] in general the research community has not been systematically involved in the implementation of their own findings and may not be well equipped to do so. In the UK, the NHS R&D Programme has made an important start by seeking views about priorities for research through a broad consultation process,[5] but better methods of involving users of research are needed to ensure that research

---

Box 1.3   Potential barriers to change may include:

Practice environment

- Limitations of time
- Practice organisation, e.g. lack of disease registers or mechanisms to monitor repeat prescribing

Educational environment

- Inappropriate continuing education and failure to link up with programmes to promote quality of care
- Lack of incentives to participate in effective educational activities

Health care environment

- Lack of financial resources
- Lack of defined practice populations
- Health policies which promote ineffective or unproven activities
- Failure to provide practitioners with access to appropriate information

Social environment

- Influence of media on patients in creating demands/beliefs
- Impact of disadvantage on patients' access to care

Practitioner factors

- Obsolete knowledge
- Influence of opinion leaders
- Beliefs and attitudes (for example, related to previous adverse experience of innovation)

Patient factors

- Demands for care
- Perceptions/cultural beliefs about appropriate care

NB Factors which in some circumstances may be perceived as barriers to change can also be levers for change. For example, patients may influence practitioners' behaviour towards clinically effective practice by requesting interventions of proven effectiveness. Practitioners may be influenced positively by opinion leaders.

---

questions are appropriately framed and tested in relevant contexts, using interventions that can be replicated in the conditions of day-to-day practice. For example, there is little point conducting trials of a new intervention in hospital practice if virtually all treatments are carried out in primary care settings. Contextual relevance is particularly important for studies of organisation and delivery of services[25] such as stroke units, hospital-at-home schemes, and schemes for improving hospital discharge. If unaccounted for, differences in skill mix and management structures between innovative services and most providers can make it difficult for providers to have a clear view of how they should best implement findings in their own units.

4. Interaction between purchasers and providers

Purchasers as well as providers should be involved in the application of research findings to practice. Purchasers can help to create an environment that is conducive to change by ensuring that health professionals have access to information, libraries are supported financially, and continuing education and audit programmes are configured to work together to promote effective practice. Purchasers can also ensure that the organisation and delivery of services take into account the best available research evidence. However, it is also clear that the degree of purchaser influence on provider practice is limited[26] and that priority must be given to helping providers to develop the capacity to understand and use evidence.

5. Making implementation an integral part of training

For many health professionals, involvement in implementation may be far more relevant to their careers and to the development of the NHS than undertaking laboratory research, yet pressures to undertake the latter remain strong. Greater emphasis should be given to encouraging clinicians to spend time learning to use and implement research findings effectively.

6. Conclusion

Enabling health professionals to evaluate research evidence and to use it in daily practice is an important part of lifelong professional development. This requires not only changes in educational programmes but also a realignment of institutions so that management structures support changes in knowledge and the implementation of changes in procedures.

Currently, there are major structural difficulties which need to be overcome in the NHS. For example better coordination is required between education and training, clinical audit, and research and development. This should be a priority for the proposed National Institute of Clinical Excellence.[27] In addition, it has recently been suggested that financial considerations rather than potential for learning needs are affecting general practitioners' choice of continuing education courses.[28] Part of continuing education should be directed towards ensuring practitioners keep up with

7

research findings of major importance for patient care and change their practice accordingly. Continuing education activities need to take into account the evidence about the ineffectiveness of many traditional approaches. To overcome fragmentation and develop a more integrated approach for promoting the uptake of research findings, health systems need to develop coordinated mechanisms to deal with the continuing evolution of medical knowledge.

The advent of research-based information[29] for patients and growing accessibility by patients to information of variable quality through the Internet and other sources suggest potential for doctors to work as information brokers and interpreters with patients and to work in concert with user groups, a number of which have demonstrated an interest and commitment to providing quality, research-based information to their members.[31] The pace of change in knowledge is unlikely to slow and as health systems around the world struggle to reconcile such change with limited resources and rising expectations, pressure to implement findings of research more effectively and efficiently is bound to grow.

References

1 Campbell NC, Thain J, Deans HG, Ritchie LD, Rawles JM. Secondary prevention in coronary heart disease: baseline survey of provision in general practice. *BMJ* (1998);**316**: 1430–4.

2 Sudlow M, Rodgers H, Kenny R, Thomson R. Population-based study of use of anticoagulants among patients with atrial fibrillation in the community. *BMJ* (1996);**314**: 1529–30.

3 Nuffield Institute for Health, University of Leeds, NHS Centre for Reviews and Dissemination, University of York, and Royal College of Physicians Research Unit. The management of menorrhagia. *Effective Health Care Bulletin 9.* Leeds: University of Leeds, 1995.

4 Enkin M. The need for Evidence based obstetrics, Evidence Based Medicine 1996; **1**: 132–3.

5 Jones R, Lamont T, Haines A. Setting priorities for research and development in the NHS: a case study on the interface between primary and secondary care. *BMJ* 1995;**311**: 1076–80.

6 Advisory Group to the NHS Central Research and Development Committee. *Methods for the implementation of the findings of research – priorities for evaluation.* Leeds: Department of Health, 1995.

7 Buxton M, Hanney S. How can payback from health services' research be assessed? *J Health Serv Res Policy* 1995;**1**:10–18.

8 Mulrow CD. Rationale for systematic reviews. *BMJ* 1994;**309**:597–9.

9 Davis DA, Thomson MA, Oxman AD, Haynes RB. Changing physician performance: a systematic review of continuing medical education strategies. *JAMA* 1995;**274**:700–5.

10 Nuffield Institute for Health, University of Leeds, NHS Centre for Reviews and Dissemination, University of York, and Royal College of Physicians Research Unit. Implementing clinical guidelines. *Effective Health Care bulletin 8.* Leeds: University of Leeds, 1994.

11 Johnston ME, Langton KB, Haynes RB, Mathiew A. The effects of computer-based clinical decision support systems on clinician performance and patients' outcome. A critical appraisal of research. *Ann Intern Med* 1994;**120**:135–42.

12 Prescott K, Douglas HR, Lloyd M, Haines A, Rosenthal J, Watt G. General Practitioners' Awareness of and attitudes towards research-based information. *Fam Pract* 1997;**14**:320–3.

13 Cimpl K. Clinical medical librarianship: a review of the literature. *Bull Med Libr Assoc* 1985;**73**:21–8.

14 Hyde CJ. Using the evidence. A need for quantity, not quality. *Int J Assess Health Care* 1996;**12(2)**:280–7.

15 Sackett DL, Haynes RB, Rosenberg W, Haynes RB. *Evidence based medicine: how to practice and teach EBM*. London: Churchill Livingstone, 1997.

16 Evidence based Medicine Working Group. Evidence based medicine. A new approach to teaching the practice of medicine. *JAMA* 1992;**268**:2420–5.

17 Oxman A, Flotorp S. An overview of strategies to promote implementation of evidence based health care. In: Silagy C, Haines A (ed.) *Evidence Based Practice in Primary Care*. BMJ Books, 1998.

18 Grol R. Beliefs and evidence in changing clinical practice. *BMJ* 1997;**315**:418–21.

19 Mittman BS, Tonesk X, Jacobson PD. Implementing clinical practice guidelines: social influence strategies and practitioner behaviour change. *Qual Rev Bull* 1992;**18**:413–21.

20 Lidstone J. *Market planning for the pharmaceutical industry*. Aldershot: Gower, 1987.

21 Oxman A, Davis D, Haynes RB, Thomson MA. No magic bullets: a systematic review of 102 trials of interventions to help health professionals deliver services more effectively or efficiently. *Can Med Assoc J* 1995;**153**:1423–43.

22 Rogers EM. *Diffusion of innovations*. New York: Free Press, 1983.

23 Haines A, Jones R. Implementing findings of research. *BMJ* 1994;**308**:1488–92.

24 Gouws D. ed. *Case studies with a view to implementation*. Pretoria, South Africa: Human Sciences Research Council, 1994.

25 Haines A, Iliffe S. Innovations in services and the appliance of science. *BMJ* 1995;**310**:875–6.

26 Hopkins A, Solomon JK. Can contracts drive clinical care? *BMJ* 1996;**313**:477–8.

27 Secretary of State for Health. *The new NHS Modern Dependable*. The Stationery Office, London 1997.

28 Murray TS, Campbell LM. Finance, not learning needs, makes general practitioners attend courses: a database survey. *BMJ* 1997;**315**:353.

29 Stocking B. Partners in care. *Health Man* 1997;**1**:12–13.

30 Stocking B. Implementing the findings of effective care in pregnancy and childbirth. *Milbank Q* 1993;**71**:497–522.

9

2 Criteria for the implementation of research evidence in policy and practice

TREVOR A SHELDON, GORDON GUYATT, AND ANDREW HAINES

Introduction

There is increasing interest in "evidence based health care" where decisions made by health care professionals, provider management, purchasers, healthcare commissioners, the public, and policy makers consistently consider research evidence.[1-3] Purchasers, for example, should be able to influence the organisation and delivery of care, such as for cancer,[4] the organisation of stroke services,[5] and the type and content of services (such as chiropractic for back pain[6] or dilatation and curettage for menorrhagia).[7] Policy makers should ensure that policy is consistent with evidence, that the incentive structure within the health system promotes cost-effective practice, and that there is an adequate infrastructure for producing, gathering, summarising, and disseminating evidence and for monitoring changes in practice. Clinicians determine the day-to-day care patients receive in health care systems and user groups are also beginning to play an important role in influencing broad health care decisions.[8]

This chapter outlines the factors that should be considered when deciding whether to act upon, or to promote the implementation of, the findings of research.

Convincing evidence of net benefit

Evaluating the methods of primary studies

Individual research studies vary in the degree to which they are likely to mis-estimate the effectiveness of an intervention (bias). Observational

10

studies, in which investigators compare the results of groups of patients receiving different treatments according to clinicians' or patients' preferences, are susceptible to bias because the prognosis of the groups is likely to differ in unpredictable ways, leading to spuriously reduced or, more commonly, inflated treatment effects.

Rigorous randomised controlled trials, by ensuring that the groups being compared are indeed similar, greatly reduce bias.[9] As long as patients are analysed in the groups to which they are randomised, this process permits a more confident inference that the treatments offered are responsible for differences in outcome. Randomised controlled trials are useful not only for testing the effectiveness of interventions in tightly controlled clinical settings but also across a wide spectrum of health research.[10,11] Inference is further strengthened if patients, care givers, and those assessing outcomes are blind to allocation to treatment or control and if follow-up is complete.[12]

Whilst randomised controlled trials are often regarded as the gold standard for comparing the efficacy of treatments, other study designs are appropriate for evaluating other types of health care technologies and factors such as potentially harmful exposures, and indicators of prognosis.[13] Increasingly, qualitative methods are being used, for example to provide an understanding of patients' and professionals' attitudes, behaviours, situations, and their interactions.[14]

Whatever the appropriate design, practitioners will often discover that research evidence is biased or otherwise limited; for example, the investigators may have focused on inappropriate end-points, such as physiological measures, rather than outcomes of relevance to patients.[15] Particularly in evaluations of health care organisation, providers must consider whether treatment effects were really due to the putative intervention. For example, in positive randomised controlled trials evaluating stroke units, was the impact due to the organisational structure or to the greater skill or enthusiasm of those who established the unit?[5] Uncertainty about the magnitude and direction of treatment effects may be heightened by small sample sizes, leading to wide confidence intervals. Though practitioners will still need to make use of imperfect research information, new clinical policies should rarely be implemented unless clinicians find strong evidence for benefit.

Evaluating the methods of overviews of groups of studies

Systematic overviews can provide reliable summaries of data addressing targeted clinical questions, and less biased estimates of treatment effects[16] if they adhere to the criteria shown in Box 2.1.[17,18]

Box 2.1 Criteria to increase reliability of a systematic review

- Use of explicit inclusion and exclusion criteria, including specification of the population, the intervention, the outcome, and the methodological criteria for the studies they include
- Comprehensive search methods used to locate relevant studies
- Assessment of the validity of the primary studies
- Assessment of the primary studies that is reproducible and attempts to avoid bias
- Exploration of variation between the study findings
- Appropriate synthesis and, when suitable, pooling of primary studies

---

Evaluating the results of systematic overviews

A rigorous systematic overview may leave the decision maker uncertain. First, the primary studies may be methodologically weak. Second, unexplained variability between study results may leave doubt about whether to believe studies showing larger treatment effects or those showing no benefit. Third, even after pooling results across studies, small sample size may leave the confidence intervals wide. Thus the research evidence may be consistent with a large, or a negligible, treatment effect. Fourth, because of the side-effects associated with a treatment, or the cost, the trade-off between treating and not treating may be precarious. Classifications of the strength of research evidence supporting use of a particular treatment should consider each of these four issues. For example, grades of strength of evidence of treatment effectiveness have been developed on methodological grounds using the type and quality of study design and the variability of study results.[19] Thus for example, a systematic review of randomised controlled trials which show consistent results (such as trials of streptokinase for treatment of acute myocardial infarction)[3] would be regarded as higher quality evidence than a review of randomised controlled trials which show variable results (heterogeneity) without good explanation. We could further consider the precision of the estimated treatment effect and the trade-off between the benefits and risks. In making the latter assessment, we must note that many studies of efficacy, and overviews of these studies, do not provide sufficient information of the possible harm (such as side-effects) of treatments. Randomised trials are usually not large or long enough to detect rare or long-term harmful effects.[20] Large observational studies may be useful in determining the probability of harm.[21]

Putting evidence of benefit into perspective

Evidence of effectiveness does not imply that an intervention should be adopted; this depends on whether the benefit is sufficiently large relative to the risks and costs. For example, the small positive effect of beta interferon in the treatment of multiple sclerosis relative to the cost leaves implementation questionable.[22,23]

One approach to the decision to implement an intervention is to determine a threshold above which one would routinely offer treatment and below which one would not. Decision makers can consider the threshold, for example in terms of the number of patients one would need to treat to prevent a single adverse event (such as a death).[24] The threshold "number needed to treat" defines the value above which the disadvantages of treatment outweigh the benefits (and treatment may therefore be withheld) and below which the benefits outweigh the disadvantages (and treatment may therefore be offered).[25] Because treatments vary with respect to their costs and their effects on length and quality of life, each intervention would need a separate threshold "number needed to treat", which will also vary according to the values of the patient or population being offered the intervention.

Where reliable data are available, a threshold might be expressed in terms of a cost-effectiveness ratio giving the cost of achieving a unit of benefit (e.g. quality-adjusted life year, taking into account equity factors) below which an intervention is seen as worth routinely implementing. Quantitative research evidence inevitably is probabilistic and subject to various forms of uncertainty and is rarely the sole basis of decision making at governmental or the clinical level. Indeed, uncertainty is one obstacle to policy makers using research evidence.[26] Differences in people's risk averseness is one explanation for variations in decision making in the face of the same evidence. However, research evidence should play an important and arguably greater part in decision making and can provide a benchmark against which decisions may be audited.

Applicability of the research to practice settings

The decision as to whether the research evidence can or should be applied in relation to a specific patient cannot always be simply translated from the research. Results of evaluative studies are usually in the form of average effects. Patients may differ from the average, however, in ways which influence the effectiveness of the treatment (relative risk reduction) or the impact (absolute risk reduction).[27,28] Box 2.2 summarises factors which clinicians and patients should consider before applying research evidence.

13

Box 2.2   Factors to consider when applying research evidence to individual patients

- Is the relative risk reduction due to the intervention likely to be different because of the patient's physiological or clinical characteristics?
- What is the patient's absolute risk of an adverse event without intervention?
- Is there significant co-morbidity or contraindication which may reduce benefit?
- Are there social or cultural factors, for example, that might affect treatment suitability or acceptability?
- What do the patient and their family want?

The sorts of patients who participate in trials may not be typical of the types of the people for whom the treatment is potentially useful.[29] However, it is probably more appropriate to assume that research findings are generalisable across patients unless there is strong theoretical or empirical evidence to suggest that a particular patient group will respond differently.[27] There may, however, be a heterogeneity of effect across patients because of biological, social, and other differences that influence the effect of the intervention or the level of risk of an adverse outcome.[29,30] For example, beta blockers may be less effective than diuretics at reducing blood pressure in black people of African descent than in white populations.[31] Interventions are more likely to impact uniformly on the population where the situation is closer to a purely biological process in which there is low variation within the population than when many patient-specific and contextual factors intervene.[32] These issues are important when targeting "effective" treatments for disadvantaged groups with the aim of reducing inequalities in health. If, for example, smoking cessation interventions are less successful in poorer groups then an anti-smoking programme might not have the anticipated effects on equity.

In a large number of chronic conditions, including chronic pain syndromes (such as arthritis from treatment) or chronic heart or lung disease where benefit may vary widely between individual patients, single-patient randomised controlled trials (N-of-1 RCTs) may help to determine a particular patient's response to treatment.[33]

Clinicians must give particular consideration to patients in whom treatment may be contraindicated or where there is substantial co-morbidity. In the latter case, a reduction of the risk of dying from one disease might not reduce overall risk of dying because of risk of a competing cause of death.

The effect of an intervention may also vary because patients do not share the same morbidity or risk.[34] For any given level of treatment effectiveness, patients at higher levels of risk will generally experience greater levels of absolute risk reduction or impact.[30,34-36] For example, patients at high risk of death from coronary heart disease treated with cholesterol-lowering drugs will experience a greater reduction in mortality risk than those at lower risk – we might have to treat 30 high-risk patients for five years to save a life, but 300 low-risk patients.[17,37,38] Thus, what might be worth implementing in a high-risk patient may not be worth it for a lower-risk patient.[37-39]

The decision to use a treatment will also depend on patient-specific factors. Clinicians will find research studies which consider a range of important outcomes of treatment more useful than those which have only measured a few narrow clinical end-points. More qualitative research within robust quantitative study design will help practitioners and patients better apply the results of research.

Setting priorities

Implementation of research evidence is rarely widespread without concerted attempts to get results into practice.[40,41] It is impossible to promote actively the implementation of the results of all systematic reviews because of the limited capacity of health care systems to absorb new research and the investment necessary to overcome obstacles to getting research into practice.[11] These costs must be considered in relation to the likely payback in terms of health improvements. The anticipated benefits of implementation will vary according to factors such as the divergence between research evidence and current practice or policies that influence the marginal benefit of further implementation efforts.

When faced with the same evidence, different classes of decision makers may have different criteria for choosing priorities for implementation. For example, policy makers look more for societal gains in health and efficiency while for clinicians the well-being of their patients is of prime importance.[42] Formal decision analysis may be helpful for setting priorities for implementation and in applying research evidence with individual patients.[43,44]

The degree to which clinicians see even good quality research as implementable will depend on the extent to which the results conflict with professional experience and cherished beliefs. This reflects an epistemological mismatch between the sort of evidence that researchers produce and believe and the sort of evidence which practising clinicians value.[45] In many cases the implications of research evidence for policy and practice are not straightforward or obvious[46] and this ambiguity may result

15

in the same evidence giving rise to divergent conclusions and action.[47] Many clinicians and policy makers will prefer to await confirmatory evidence, depending on the perceived risks, the extent of change required, and the quality and certainty of the research results. When designing studies, investigators should think how and by whom their results will be used. The design should be sufficiently robust, the setting sufficiently similar to that in which the results are likely to be implemented, the outcomes should be relevant, and the study size large enough for the results to convince decision makers.

References

1 Davidoff F, Haynes RB, Sackett D, Smith R. Evidence based medicine [editorial]. *BMJ* 1995;**310**:1122–6.
2 Guyatt GH. Evidence based medicine [editorial]. *ACP J Club* 1991;A–16.
3 Antman EM, Lau J, Kupelnick B, Mosteller F, Chalmers TC. A comparison of the results of controlled trials and recommendations of clinical experts. Treatments for myocardial infarction. *JAMA* 1992;**268**:240–8.
4 *NHS Executive guidance for purchasers: Improving outcomes in breast cancer – the manual* (96CC0021). London: Department of Health, 1996.
5 Stroke Unit Trialists' Collaboration. A systematic review of specialist multidisciplinary (stroke unit) care for stroke in patients. In: Warlow C, van Gijn J, Sandercock P. ed. *Stroke module of the Cochrane Database of Systematic Reviews*. London: BMJ Publishing Group, 1997.
6 Shekelle P. *Spinal manipulation and mobilisation for low back pain.* Paper presented at the International Forum for Primary Care Research on Low Back Pain, Seattle, October 1995.
7 NHS Centre for Reviews and Dissemination; University of York. Management of menorrhagia. *Effective Health Care Bulletin* 1995;**1**(9).
8 Entwistle V, Sheldon TA, Sowden A, Watt I. Evidence-informed patient choice: issues of involving patients in decisions about health care technologies. *Int J Tech Assess Health Care.* 1998; (in press).
9 Schultz K, Chalmers I, Haynes RJ, Altman DG. Empirical evidence of bias. Dimensions of methodological quality associated with estimates of treatment effects in controlled clinical trials. *JAMA* 1995;**273**:408–12.
10 Green SB. The eating patterns study – the importance of practical randomized trials in communities. *Am J Public Health* 1997;**87**:541–3.
11 Bauman KE. The effectiveness of family planning programs evaluated with true experimental designs. *Am J Public Health* 1997;**87**:666–9.
12 Guyatt GH, Sackett DL, Cook DJ for the evidence based medicine working group. Users' guide to the medical literature. II. How to use an article about therapy or prevention. Part A – Are the results valid? *JAMA* 1993;**270**:2598–601.
13 Laupacis A, Wells G, Richardson WS, Tugwell P for the evidence based medicine working group. Users' guides to the medical literature. V. How to use an article about prognosis. *JAMA* 1994;**272**:234–7.
14 Mays N, Pope C. *Qualitative research in health care.* London: BMJ Publishing Group, 1996.
15 Gotzsche PC, Liberati A, Torri V, Rossetti L. Beware of surrogate end-points. *Int J Tech Assess Health Care* 1996;**12**:238–46.
16 Chalmers I, Altman D. *Systematic reviews.* London: BMJ Publishing Group, 1995.
17 Oxman AD, Cook DJ, Guyatt GH for the evidence based medicine working group. Users' guide to the medical literature. VI. How to use an overview. *JAMA* 1993;**272**:1367–71.

18 *Undertaking systematic reviews of research on effectiveness. CRD guidelines for those carrying out or commissioning reviews.* CRD Report 4. University of York: NHS Centre for Reviews and Dissemination, 1996.

19 Liddle J, Williamson M, Irwig L. *Method for evaluating research and guidelines evidence.* Sydney: NSW Health Department, 1996.

20 Levine M, Walter S, Lee H, Haines T, Holbrook A, Moyer V for the evidence based medicine working group. Users' guides to the medical literature. IV. How to use an article about harm. *JAMA* 1994;**271**:1615–19.

21 Palareti G, Leali N, Coccher S, *et al.* Bleeding complications of oral anticoagulant treatment: an inception-cohort, prospective collaborative study (ISCOAT). *Lancet* 1996: **348**;423–8.

22 Walley T, Barton S. A purchaser perspective of managing new drugs: interferon beta as a case study. *BMJ* 1995;**311**:796–9.

23 Rous E, Coppel A, Haworth J, Noyce S. A purchaser experience of managing new expensive drugs: interferon beta. *BMJ* 1996;**313**:1195–6.

24 Cook RJ, Sackett DL, The number needed to treat – a clinically useful measure of treatment. *BMJ* 1995;**310**:452–4.

25 Guyatt GH, Sackett DL, Sinclair JC *et al.* Users' guide to the medical literature. IX. A method for grading health care recommendations. *JAMA* 1995;**274**:1800–4.

26 Hammond K, Mumpower J, Dennis RL, Fitch S, Crumpacker W. Fundamental obstacles to the use of scientific information in public policy making. *Technological Forecasting and Social Change* 1983;**24**:287–97.

27 Davis CE. Generalizing from clinical trials. *Controlled Clinical Trials* 1994;**15**:11–14.

28 Wittes RE. Problems in the medical interpretation of overviews. *Stats in Med* 1987;**6**: 269–76.

29 Pearson TA, Myers M. Treatment of hypercholesterolemia in women: equality, effectiveness, and extrapolation of evidence. *JAMA* 1997;**277**:1320–1.

30 Bailey KR. Generalizing the results of randomized clinical trials. *Controlled Clinical Trials* 1994;**15**:15–23.

31 Veterans Administration Cooperative Study Group. Comparison of propranolol and hydrochlorothiazide for the initial treatment of hypertension. 1: Results of short-term titration with emphasis on racial differences in response. *JAMA* 1982;**248**:1996 2003.

32 Cowan CD, Wittes J. Intercept studies, clinical trials, and cluster experiments: to whom can we extrapolate? *Controlled Clinical Trials* 1994;**15**:24–9

33 Mahon J, Laupacis A, Donner A, Wood T. Randomised study of N-of-1 trials versus standard practice. *BMJ* 1996;**312**:1069–74.

34 Davey Smith G, Eggar M. Who benefits from medical interventions? *BMJ* 1993;**308**: 72–4.

35 Glasziou PP, Irwig LM. An evidence based approach to individualising treatment. *BMJ* 1995;**311**:356–9.

36 Oxman AD, Guyatt GH. A consumer's guide to subgroup analysis. *Ann Intern Med* 1992; **116**;78–84.

37 Davey Smith G, Song F, Sheldon TA. Cholesterol lowering and mortality: the importance of considering initial level of risk. *BMJ* 1993;**306**:1367–73.

38 Marchioli R, Marfisi RM, Carinci F, Tognoni G. Meta-analysis, clinical trials, and transferability of research results into practice. *Arch Intern Med* 1996;**156**:1158–72.

39 Ramsey LE, Haq IU, Jackson PR, Yeo WW, Pickin DM, Payne N. Targeting lipid-lowering drug therapy for primary prevention of coronary disease: an updated Sheffield table. *Lancet* 1996;**348**:387–8.

40 Oxman A, Davis D, Haynes RB, Thomson MA. No magic bullets: a systematic review of 102 trials of interventions to help health professionals deliver services more effectively and efficiently. *Can Med Assoc J* 1995;**153**:1423–43.

41 Haines A, Jones R. Implementing findings of research. *BMJ* 1994;**308**:1488–92.

42 Diamond GA, Denton TA. Alternative perspectives on the biased foundation of medical technology assessment. *Ann Intern Med* 1993;**118**:455–64.

43 Thornton JG, Lilford RJ. Decision analysis for managers. *BMJ* 1995;**310**:791–4.

44 Lilford RJ, Thornton JG. Decision logic in medical practice. *J Royal Coll Phys* 1992;**26**: 400–12.

45 Tanenbaum SJ. Knowing and acting in medical practice: the epistemological politics of outcomes research. *J Health Politics and Law* 1994;**19**:27–44.
46 Naylor CD. Grey zones of clinical practice: some limits to evidence based medicine. *Lancet* 1995;**345**:840–2.
47 Tanenbaum SJ. "Medical effectiveness" in Canadian and US health policy: the comparative politics of inferential ambiguity. *Health Serv Res* 1996;**31**:517–32.

3 Sources of information on clinical effectiveness and methods of dissemination

JULIE GLANVILLE, MARGARET HAINES, AND IONE AUSTON

Introduction

There is increasing pressure on health care professionals to ensure that their practice is based on evidence from good quality research such as well-conducted randomised controlled trials or preferably systematic reviews of these and other research designs. This pressure comes from various directions. The evidence based health care movement is encouraging a questioning and reflective approach to clinical practice alongside an emphasis on lifelong learning. This relies on good access to research-based evidence. Governments are encouraging the development of evidence based medicine as they see its advantages in terms of improved efficiency in the delivery of health care through identification of effective treatments.[1,2] In addition there are indications that legal decisions may start to take account of adherence to research evidence and clinical guidelines.[3,4] Another incentive for clinicians to be more aware of research may come from better informed consumers. Being able to access information on clinical effectiveness in order to improve quality of care and to stay well informed on specialist areas of health care looks set to become a basic skill for the clinician. This chapter examines the issues of access to research-based evidence from three perspectives:

(1) resources that are already available for clinicians to use
(2) further strategies for finding and filtering information
(3) improvements to dissemination practices so that relevant material can be more easily identified.

What evidence based information is currently available?

In the 1990s great progress has been made in making evidence from research more easily available. In part this has been achieved through the development of programmes of health technology assessments and, in particular, the growth of systematic reviews. Systematic reviews evaluate the available primary evidence and indicate the effectiveness of particular interventions. They necessarily take some time to complete, but already a useful compilation of reviews is available in the Cochrane Library and reports have been appearing from technology assessment agencies such as the Agency for Health Care Policy and Research (AHCPR) in the United States and the English Department of Health's Health Technology Assessment Programme. The publications and databases listed in Box 3.1 present evidence on effectiveness, often in a summarised or digested form suitable for the busy clinician or policy maker. However, key problems remain: how to increase awareness of what information is available and how to provide clinicians with information at the time that they need it.

Collections of systematic reviews and critical appraisals of primary research provide valuable access to evaluated research. Inevitably, the proliferation of these collections is creating its own information explosion which needs to be speedily addressed. There is currently no single comprehensive index to all the material described in Box 3.1 so several searches in paper and electronic services may be required to locate relevant information. It may also be necessary to obtain copies of the original publication. These factors create disincentives to use to which information technology may eventually provide a more streamlined solution in the form of World Wide Web-type interfaces that provide links to a range of quality-filtered, evaluated, evidence based information services as well as access to the full text of publications. Biomednet is one model of service, offering a range of full text resources alongside free MEDLINE as well as providing discussion facilities and "meeting rooms". It is beginning to offer a quality-filtering approach by highlighting significant papers which have been cited and evaluated by expert reviewers.[5]

Most of the resources in Box 3.1 provide evaluated and filtered information, i.e. they highlight the best quality studies from the mass of available literature. However, research-based answers to many effectiveness questions are not yet available in such time-saving, value-added forms. Searchers may still need to search indexes and abstracts of the published literature. For several years it has been possible for clinicians to search MEDLINE themselves using software such as Grateful Med and its World Wide Web interface, Internet Grateful Med. This has provided access to a mass of peer-reviewed but largely unsynthesized and unevaluated studies. There are now tools which can help searchers to identify the types of

Box 3.1 Selected resources providing summaries or assessments of the effectiveness of interventions

The Cochrane Library

A collection of databases, including the full text of Cochrane Collaboration Reviews, critical commentaries on selected quality-assessed systematic reviews produced by the NHS Centre for Reviews and Dissemination, and brief details of more than 150 000 randomised controlled trials. Details: Update Software, Summertown Pavillion, Middle Way, Summertown, Oxford OX2 7LG. For details of Internet access see URLs: http://www.medlib.com and http://www.hcn.net.au/.

Agency for Health Care Policy and Research (AHCPR) clinical guidelines

A series of clinical guidelines based on thorough reviews of the research evidence. AHCPR is now focusing on producing evidence reports as well as working with the American Medical Association and the American Association of Health Plans on an on-line practice guidelines clearing-house that will have an electronic mailing list feature to keep users informed about guideline implementation.
Details: URL: http://text.nlm.nih.gov/ and http://www.ahcpr.gov/.

Best Evidence database

Brings together abstracts (published in *ACP Journal Club* and *Evidence based Medicine*) of quality-assessed primary and review articles with a commentary by clinical experts.
Details: (1) Website URL: http://hiru.hirunet.mcmaster.ca/acpjc;
(2) A CD-ROM is available from BMJ Publishing, BMA House, Tavistock Square, London WC1H 9JR.

Effective Health Care Bulletins

Reports of systematic reviews presented in a readable and accessible format. Produced by the NHS Centre for Reviews and Dissemination.
Details: Subscriptions Department, Pearson Professional, PO Box 77, Fourth Avenue, Harlow CM19 5BQ.

Guide to clinical preventive services, 2nd edn. Report of the US Preventive Services Task Force

Evidence based recommendations on preventive services.
Details: URL: http://text.nlm.nih.gov/.

Canadian guide to clinical preventive health care

Evidence based recommendations on preventive services.
Details: Ottawa: Health Canada, 1994.

continued

Box 3.1 *continued*

Bandolier

UK newsletter alerting readers to key evidence about health care effectiveness.
Details: URL: http://www.jr2.ox.ac.uk/Bandolier.

Drug and Therapeutics Bulletin

Independent assessments of drugs and other modes of treatment.
Details: Consumers' Association, Castlemead, Gascoyne Way, Hertford SG14 1LH. URL: http://www.which.net/nonsub/pubs/dtb/intro.html.

Effectiveness Matters

Summaries of published research on a single topic pointing out clear effectiveness messages.
Details: NHS Centre for Reviews and Dissemination, University of York, York YO1 5DD. URL: http://www.york.ac.uk/inst.ord.

MeReC Bulletin

Summary reviews of major new drugs aimed at GPs and addressing issues of effectiveness, safety, appropriateness, acceptability, and cost.
Details: Medicines Resource Centre, Hamilton House, 24 Pall Mall, Liverpool L3 6AL.

NHS Economic Evaluation database

Critical assessments of published economic evaluations, produced by the NHS Centre for Reviews and Dissemination.
Details: URL: http://www.york.ac.uk/inst/crd.

---

studies that are more likely to provide high quality information on clinical effectiveness, such as systematic reviews or randomised controlled trials.[6,7] Once the original papers have been obtained there are checklists which, complemented by critical appraisal skills training, can be used to assess the rigour and validity of such studies.[8–10]

Although MEDLINE is a rich resource, increasingly access is required to a wider range of material than it presently indexes. The US National Library of Medicine and the American Hospital Association have recently launched HealthSTAR which seeks to provide expanded access to both non-clinical and non-journal information.[11] The National Library of Medicine has recently announced free access to MEDLINE and HealthSTAR through Internet Grateful Med and free access to MEDLINE through the PubMed interface.[12] Other databases covering specific clinical areas, specific types of publication, and non-English material also need to be more widely explored. Tools such as search strategies and single interfaces, such as Internet Grateful Med, are required that will enhance access to a range of such databases.

Other strategies for finding and filtering information

Training and practice are required to search information services and navigate the Internet effectively, but other options are available which may help the individual cope with the challenges of finding information. Locating, appraising, and exploiting subject resources, both print and electronic, has typically been the role of the librarian or information professional. Increasingly, clinicians may find that librarians can not only help them locate information to answer a particular issue but can also help to keep them up to date by presenting selections of key new evidence in the form of paper or electronic current awareness bulletins.

The value of library and information support has been demonstrated on both sides of the Atlantic. Librarians are often more effective than physicians, particularly trained librarians compared to untrained physicians, in quality filtering of the literature.[13] Other American studies have shown that library support not only contributes to lower patient costs through decreased admissions, length of stay, and procedures but also contributes to higher quality of care in terms of patient advice, improved decision making, and time saving.[14,15] A similar study in the UK also demonstrated the positive impact of library services on the continuing education of hospital doctors.[16]

Not all clinicians have the time to visit libraries and new models have emerged for delivering library support directly to the hospital wards and departments.[17,18] In the United States, the National Network of Libraries of Medicine provide outreach services to general practitioners (and, more recently, to public health professionals) and in the UK the British Medical Association Library also offers an electronic outreach service to members.[19,20] In the UK, the Oxford Primary Care Sharing the Evidence (PRISE) project is looking at another model whereby GPs' computers are linked into a central information server computer which provides a range of useful databases and can also request librarians to follow up particular questions in more detail.[21] Librarians are increasingly asked to provide information skills training as part of courses in evidence based medicine for NHS staff. The development of primary care-based services presents a challenge to librarians to become better trained to deal with a wide range of clinician enquiries, to evaluate and synthesise the available evidence, and to present selected information through innovative outreach delivery systems. Clearly, initiatives such as the Oxford Health Libraries' training programme "Librarian of the Twenty-First Century" is a model for other library networks.[22] Similar initiatives under development in the US include the National Information Center on Health Services Research and Health Care Technology (NICHSR) Web-based training materials[23] and National Library of Medicine grants to seven institutions to provide health sciences librarian education and training planning.

How can researchers, publishers, and information providers improve dissemination?

This chapter has looked at strategies to locate research-based information. For information to be accessible it must also be packaged and published in formats that promote easy identification and encourage use. Evidence based information is becoming easier to spot: structured abstracts attached to journal articles are making it easier to identify the methodology and so potentially the reliability of the study. Innovations such as the *British Medical Journal*'s key messages box make it easier to identify the key points to be drawn from the research. Journal editors have an important role in encouraging informative abstracts and ensuring that researchers' conclusions are supported by a paper's results. However, the benefits of clearer labelling may be undermined if current "buzzwords" such as "effective" and "evidence based" are adopted and used incorrectly or inaccurately: previously useful labels may become unhelpful.

Bodies producing policy and clinical recommendations, including guidelines, are finding it necessary to make them more explicitly evidence based, both in using the available research evidence and in stating the level of evidence on which the guidance is based.[24,25] It would be easier to assess guidelines if the evidence base was as clearly stated as possible, for example a statement on the front cover: "This guideline is based on a Cochrane review." This sort of evidence-level "Kitemark" could be a time-saving innovation. The Guideline Appraisal Project of the Health Information Research Unit at McMaster University is an example of efforts to help practitioners to identify and critically appraise clinical guidelines, and to determine their applicability in local practice.[26]

Information from research needs to be presented in appropriate forms for its target audience. The AHCPR guidelines have shown how information can be packaged in different ways for different groups of users by using three levels of publication: a detailed report of the review with a full exposition of the research evidence, a briefer guideline for the clinician, and a leaflet for the patient. In the UK, the Informed Choice leaflets have shown how different leaflets aimed at pregnant women and their professional carers can be produced, based on evidence taken where possible from Cochrane reviews.[27,28]

Improving timely access to information is only one aspect of the implementation of research-based information. Simply presenting research evidence to the clinician is often not sufficient to ensure its incorporation into practice. Government directives and direct incentives can increase swift uptake and sometimes powerful research findings will have an immediate effect: swift changes in practice followed the publication of research findings that sleeping position can affect mortality from sudden infant death syndrome.[29,30] However, even when findings are packaged, summarised, and made relevant to clinicians, further action is needed to ensure their implementation.

A complex set of factors influence the uptake of research findings and a variety of dissemination methods need to be employed to encourage informed changes in practice.[31] Much research on effective implementation is currently underway, but part of the answer could be a nationally coordinated strategy to disseminate and promote important evidence appearing from research and systematic reviews to health care professionals. National campaigns with coordinated distribution of information packs, briefings, videos, and information points for important research findings might also assist in the wider adoption of informed changes in practice. Such national campaigns would need to be complemented by a variety of other activities at a local level.[32] Local implementation strategies, continuing education and patient education programmes, and library and information outreach services could be coordinated to ensure that key published research evidence is not only accessible but also acted upon.

Acknowledgements

Helpful comments on this paper were received from Olwen Jones, Susan Mottram, Ian Watt, Trevor Sheldon, and Andrew Jones.

References

1 *Priorities and planning guidance for the NHS: 1997/98.* Leeds: Department of Health, NHS Executive, 1996.
2 Glasziou PP. Support for trials of promising medications through the Pharmaceutical Benefits Scheme. A proposal for a new authority category. *Med J Aust* 1995;**162**:33–6.
3 Stern K. Clinical guidelines and negligence liability. In: Deighan M, Hitch S. ed. *Clinical effectiveness from guidelines to cost-effective practice.* Brentwood: Earlybrave Publications, 1995:
4 Doctors in the dock. *Economist* 1995;**Aug 19**:23–4.
5 URL: http://biomednet.com/.
6 Dickersin K, Scherer R, Lefebvre C. Identifying relevant studies for systematic reviews. *BMJ* 1994;**309**:1286–91.
7 McKibbon KA, Wilczynski NL, Walker-Dilks CJ. How to search for and find evidence about therapy. *Evidence based Med* 1996;**1**(3):70–2.
8 Oxman AD. Check-lists for review articles. *BMJ* 1994;**309**:648–51.
9 Hayward RS, Wilson MC, Tunis SR, Bass EB, Guyatt GH. How to use clinical practice guidelines. A. Are the recommendations valid? *JAMA* 1995;**274**:570–4.

25

10 Wilson MC, Hayward RS, Tunis SR, Bass EB, Guyatt GH. How to use clinical practice guidelines. B. What are the results and will they help me in caring for my patients? *JAMA* 1995;**274**:1630–2.

11 HealthSTAR [bibliographic database–CD-ROM and on-line]. (1975–present). National Library of Medicine (producer).

12 URL: http://www.nlm.nih.gov/databases/freemedl.html.

13 Fuller AB, Wessel CB, Ginn DS, Martin TP. Quality filtering of the clinical literature by librarians and physicians. *Bull Med Libr Assoc* 1993;**81**:38–43.

14 Marshall, JG. The impact of the hospital library on clinical decision making: the Rochester Study. *Bull Med Libr Assoc* 1992;**80**:169–78.

15 Klein MS, Ross FV, Adams DL, Gilbert CM. Effects of on-line literature searching on length of stay and patient care costs. *Acad Med* 1994;**69**(6):489–95.

16 Urquhart CJ, Hepworth JB. *The value to clinical decision making of information supplied by NHS library and information services.* British Library R&D Report 6205. London: The British Library, 1995.

17 Cimpl K. Clinical medical librarianship: a review of the literature. *Bull Med Libr Assoc* 1985;**73**:21–8.

18 Schatz CA, Whitehead SE. "Librarian for hire": contracting a librarian's services to external departments. *Bull Med Libr Assoc* 1995;**83**:469–72.

19 Wallingford KT, Ruffin AB, Ginter KA, *et al.* Outreach activities of the National Library of Medicine: a five-year review. *Bull Med Libr Assoc* 1996;**84**:April supplement.

20 Rowlands JK, Forrester WH, McSean T. British Medical Association Library free MEDLINE service: survey of members taking part in an initial pilot project. *Bull Med Libr Assoc* 1996;**84**:116–21.

21 URL: http://wwwlib.jr2.ox.ac.uk/prise/.

22 Palmer J, Streatfield, D. Good diagnosis for the twenty-first century. *Libr Assoc Rec* 1995; **97**:153–4.

23 URL: http://www.nlm.nih.gov/nichsr.

24 Scottish Intercollegiate Guidelines Network. *Clinical guidelines: criteria for appraisal for national use.* Edinburgh: SIGN, 1995.

25 NHS Executive. *Improving outcomes in breast cancer: the research evidence.* London: Department of Health, 1996.

26 URL: http://hiru.mcmaster.ca/cpg/.

27 *Informed choice* [leaflets]. Bristol: Midwives Information and Resource Service, 1995.

28 Oliver S, Rajan L, Turner H, Oakley A. A pilot study of "*Informed Choice*" leaflets on positions in labour and routine ultrasound. University of York: NHS Centre for Reviews and Dissemination, 1996.

29 Spiers PS, Guntheroth WG. Recommendations to avoid the prone sleeping position and recent statistics for sudden infant death syndrome in the United States. *Arch Pediatr Adolesc Med* 1994;**148**(2):141–6.

30 Hilley CM, Morley CJ. Evaluation of government's campaign to reduce risk of cot death. *BMJ* 1994;**309**:703–4.

31 Deykin D, Haines A. Promoting the use of research findings. In: Peckham M, Smith R. ed. *Scientific basis for health services.* London: BMJ Publishing Group, 1996.

32 Davis DA, Thomson MA, Oxman AD, Haynes RB. Changing physician performance: a systematic review of the effect of continuing medical education strategies. *JAMA* 1995; **274**(9):700–5.

4 Closing the gap between research and practice: an overview of systematic reviews of interventions to promote implementation of research findings by health care professionals

LISA BERO, ROBERTO GRILLI, JEREMY GRIMSHAW, EMMA HARVEY, ANDY OXMAN, AND MARY ANN THOMSON

ON BEHALF OF THE COCHRANE EFFECTIVE PRACTICE AND ORGANISATION OF CARE GROUP

Introduction

Despite the considerable resources spent on clinical research, relatively little attention has been paid to ensuring that the findings of research are acted upon in routine clinical practice.[1] There are many different interventions to promote professional behavioural change that could be used to implement research findings (Box 4.1). Disentangling the effects of interventions from the influence of contextual factors is difficult when interpreting the results of individual behavioural change trials.[2] Nevertheless, systematic reviews of rigorous evaluations provide the best evidence of the effectiveness of different behavioural change strategies.[3,4] In this chapter, we undertake an overview of systematic reviews of different dissemination and implementation interventions to identify evidence of effectiveness of different strategies and to assess the quality of systematic reviews in this area.

27

Methods

Inclusion criteria

We sought any systematic review of interventions to improve professional performance that reported explicit selection criteria and in which the main outcomes considered were changes in professional performance or patient outcomes. Reviews that did not report explicit selection criteria, systematic reviews focusing on the methodological quality of published studies, published bibliographies, bibliographic databases, and registers of projects on dissemination activities were excluded. Where systematic reviews had been updated, we only considered the most recently published review. For example, the *Effective Health Care Bulletin* on implementing clinical guidelines[5] superseded the previous review by Grimshaw and Russell.[6]

Identification of systematic reviews

We searched MEDLINE between 1966 and June 1995 using a strategy developed in collaboration with the NHS Centre for Reviews and Dissemination. The search identified 1139 references. Overall, we identified 18 reviews fulfilling our inclusion criteria. No reviews from the Cochrane Effective Practice and Organisation of Care Module had been published during this time period. In addition, we searched the Database of Abstracts of Research Effectiveness (DARE)[7] but did not identify any other review which fulfilled our inclusion criteria.

Quality assessment and data extraction

Two reviewers independently assessed the quality of identified reviews and extracted data about the focus, inclusion criteria, main results, and conclusions of each review. A previously validated check-list (including nine criteria scored as *done, partially done, and not done*. Major disagreements between reviewers were resolved by consensus.

Results

Reviews identified

We identified 18 broad reviews focusing on: *broad strategies* (for example, dissemination and implementation of guidelines,[5,10–12] continuing medical

28

education,[13,14] *particular strategies* (for example, audit and feedback;[15,16] computerised decision support;[17,18] multifaceted interventions,[19] *particular target audiences* (for example, nurses;[20] primary care,[21] and *particular problem areas or types of behaviour* (for example, diagnostic testing;[16] prescribing;[22] aspects of preventive care;[16,23–25] and training professionals in smoking cessation techniques[26]). Detailed descriptions of the reviews are published elsewhere. No reviews published before 1987 were identified. None of the reviews explicitly addressed the cost-effectiveness of different behaviour change strategies.

Quality assessment

There was a lack of a common approach adopted within the reviews to categorise interventions and potential confounding factors. The inclusion criteria and methods used in these reviews varied considerably. Interventions were frequently classified differently by reviews. For example, Lomas and colleagues[27] evaluated the impact of provincial guidelines to reduce caesarian section rates. The *Effective Health Care Bulletin*[5] classified the intervention as a "Consensus Development Conference [producing] external provincial guidelines [which were] distributed by publication in professional journals and mailing to targeted clinicians, [with] no further attempt at implementation", whereas the review by Mugford and colleagues[15] classified the intervention as "information feedback on operative proceedures".

Common methodological problems included: failure to adequately report criteria for selecting studies to include in the review; failure to avoid bias in the selection of studies; failure to adequately report criteria to assess validity; and failure to apply criteria to assess validity to the selected studies. Overall, 42% (68/162) criteria were reported as done, 49.4% (80/162) partially done, and 8.6% (14/162) not done whilst the mean summary score was 4.13 (range 2–6, median 3.75, mode 3). Encouragingly, more recently published reviews appeared to be of better quality. Only 20.4% (11/54) criteria were scored as done with a mean summary score of 3.0 for studies published between 1988 and 1991 (n=6), compared with 51.9% (56/108) criteria scored as done with a mean summary score of 4.7 for reviews published after 1991 (n=12).

Only five reviews[13,18,20,24,26] attempted formal meta-analysis of the results of the identified studies. The appropriateness of meta-analysis in three of these reviews is uncertain and should be considered exploratory at best, given the broad focus and heterogeneity of the included studies with respect to the types of interventions, the targeted behaviours, contextual factors, and other research factors.[2]

Results of reviews

A number of consistent themes are identified by the systematic reviews (Box 4.1). Most of the reviews identified modest improvements in performance following interventions. However, passive dissemination of information by itself was generally ineffective in altering physician practices, no matter how important the issue or how valid the assessment methods.[5,10,12,14,22] Computerised decision support and remainders systems have led to improvements in physician performance in drug dosage decisions, provision of preventive care, and general clinical management of patients but not diagnosis across a variety of settings and conditions.[16–19,21,24,25] Educational outreach visits have resulted in improvements in prescribing decisions in North American settings.[5,14] Patient-mediated interventions appear to improve provision of preventive care in North American settings (where baseline performance is often very low).[14] Audit and feedback appear to reduce inappropriate diagnostic test ordering and prescribing practices.[15,16,19] Multifaceted interventions appear to be more effective than single interventions.[14,19] There is insufficient evidence to assess the effectiveness of some interventions, for example the identification and recruitment of local opinion leaders.[5]

Few reviews attempted explicitly to link their findings to theories of behaviour change. The difficulties associated with this are illustrated in the review by Davis and colleagues[14] which observed that the results of the overview supported several different theories of behaviour change.

Availability and quality of primary studies

This overview also allows the opportunity to estimate the availability and quality of primary research in an area. Identification of published behavioural change studies is difficult because they are poorly indexed and scattered across generalist and specialist journals. Nevertheless, two reviews provided an indication of the extent of research in this area: Oxman and colleagues[12] identified 102 randomised or quasi-randomised controlled trials of interventions to improve professional practice. The *Effective Health Care Bulletin*[5] on implementing clinical guidelines identified 91 rigorous studies (including 63 randomised or quasi-randomised controlled trials and 28 controlled or strengthened before and after studies). Even though these studies fulfilled the criteria for inclusion in the systematic reviews, some are methodologically flawed with potentially major threats to internal or external validity. Many studies randomised professionals or groups of professionals (cluster randomisation) but analysed the results by patient, resulting in a possible overestimation of the statistical significance of the observed effects (unit of analysis error).[28] Given the small to moderate size

30

Box 4.1   Interventions to promote professional behavioural change

Consistently Effective

Educational outreach visits (for prescribing in North American settings)
Reminders (manual or computerised)
Multifaceted interventions – a combination that includes two or more of the following: audit and feedback, reminders, local consensus process, marketing
Interactive educational meetings – Participation of health care providers in workshops that include discussion or practice

Mixed Effects

Audit and feedback – Any summary of clinical performance
Local opinion leaders – Use of providers nominated by their colleagues as 'educationally influential'
Local consensus process – Inclusion of participating providers in discussion to ensure that they agreed that the chosen clinical problem was important and the approach to managing the problem was appropriate
Patient mediated interventions – Any intervention aimed at changing the performance of health care providers where specific information was sought from or given to patients

Little or No Effect

Educational materials – Distribution of published or printed recommendations for clinical care, including clinical practice guidelines, audio-visual materials and electronic publications
Didactic educational meetings – Lectures

---

of the observed effects, this could lead to false conclusions of statistical significance in both meta-analyses and qualitative analyses. Few studies attempted to undertake any form of economic analysis.

Given the importance of implementing the results of sound research and problems related to generalisability across different health care settings, there are relatively few studies of individual professional behaviour change interventions. The review by Oxman and colleagues[12] identified 12 studies of educational materials, 17 of conferences, four of outreach visits, six of local opinion leaders, 10 of patient mediated interventions, 33 of audit and feedback, 53 of reminders, two of marketing, eight of local consensus processes, and 15 of multifaceted interventions. Few studies compared the relative effectiveness of different strategies: only 22 out of 91 studies reviewed in the *Effective Health Care Bulletin* allowed comparisons of different strategies.[5] A further limitation of the evidence about individual

31

types of intervention is that the research is often conducted by limited numbers of research groups in specific settings. The generalisability of these findings to other settings is uncertain given the marked differences in undergraduate and postgraduate education, organisation of health care, societal values and culture, and likely system incentives and barriers to change. Most of the published studies were conducted in North America and only 14 of 91 studies reviewed in the *Effective Health Care Bulletin* had been conducted in European settings.[5]

Discussion

This overview suggests that there is increasing primary and secondary research in this area. The quality of both primary and secondary research is variable and could be improved. However, it is striking how little is currently known about the effectiveness and cost-effectiveness of interventions aiming to achieve changes in practice or the delivery of health care. The reviews suggest that the passive dissemination of information (for example, publication of consensus conferences in professional journals or mailing educational materials) is generally ineffective and at best resulted only in very small effects on physician practice. However, these probably represent the most common approaches adopted by researchers, professional bodies, and local purchaser and provider organisations. Specific strategies to implement research-based recommendations appear necessary to ensure practice change, and existing studies suggest that more intensive efforts to alter practice are generally more successful.

At the service level, greater attention needs to be given to coordinating active dissemination and implementation strategies to ensure the uptake of research findings. At present, the choice of intervention should be guided by the characteristics of the message[11] and recognition of external barriers to change[14] and the preparedness to change of the targeted clinicians.[29] Local groups need to be aware of the results of implementation research, develop expertise in the principles of management of change, and accept the need for local experimentation.

Given the paucity of evidence, it is vital that dissemination and implementation activities should be rigorously evaluated whenever possible. Studies evaluating a single intervention provide little new information about the relative effectiveness and cost-effectiveness of different interventions in different settings. Greater emphasis should be given to studies which evaluate two or more interventions in a specific setting or help clarify the circumstances that are likely to modify the effectiveness of an intervention. Economic evaluation should be considered an integral component of research in this area. Researchers should have greater awareness of the issues related to cluster randomisation and ensure that studies have adequate power and are analysed using appropriate methods.[30]

The NHS R&D Programme on Evaluating Methods to Promote the Implementation of R&D is a major initiative which will contribute substantially to our knowledge in this area.[31] However, the research issues cut across national and cultural differences in the practice and financing of health care. Moreover, the scope of these issues is such that no individual country's health services research programme alone can examine them in a comprehensive way. This suggests the potential benefits of international collaboration and cooperation in this area with due regard to cultural factors which may influence the implementation process through the beliefs and perceptions of the public, patients, health care professionals, and policy makers.

The results of primary research should be systematically reviewed to identify promising implementation techniques and areas where more research is required.[3] Undertaking reviews in this area is difficult because of the complexity inherent in the interventions, variability in methods used, and the difficulty of generalising study findings across health care settings.[2] The Cochrane Effective Practice and Organisation of Care Group is helping to meet the need for systematic reviews of current best evidence of CME, quality assurance, and other growing interventions that affect professional practice. A growing number of these reviews are being published and updated in the Cochrane Database of Systematic Reviews.[4,32]

Acknowledgements

This chapter is based upon a briefing paper prepared by the authors for the Advisory Group on the NHS R&D Programme on Evaluating Methods to Promote the Implementation of R&D. This work was partly funded by the EC-funded EUR ASSESS project. The Cochrane Collaboration on Effective Professional Practice is funded by the following Regional Research and Development directorates: North Thames, South Thames, Trent, West Midlands, North West, and South and West in the United Kingdom and by the Norwegian Research Council and Ministry of Health and Social Affairs in Norway. The Health Services Research Unit is funded by the Chief Scientist's Office of the Scottish Office Home and Health Department. However, the views expressed are those of the authors and not necessarily the funding bodies.

References

1 Eddy DM. Clinical policies and the quality of clinical practice. *New Engl J Med* 1982; **307**:343–7.

2 Grimshaw JM, Freemantle N, Langhorne P, Song F. *Complexity and systematic reviews.* Report to the US Congress of Technology Assessment. Washington DC: Office of Technology Assessment, 1995.

3 Mulrow CD. Rationale for systematic reviews. *BMJ* 1994;**309**:597–9.

4 Bero L, Grilli R, Grimshaw JM, Oxman AD. ed. The Cochrane Collaboration on Effective Professional Practice Module of The Cochrane Database of Systematic Reviews, Cochrane Library. 4th edn. London: BMJ Publishing Group, 1997.

5 *Implementing clinical guidelines. Can guidelines be used to improve clinical practice? Effective Health Care Bulletin No 8.* Leeds: University of Leeds, 1994.

6 Grimshaw JM, Russell IT. Effect of clinical guidelines on medical practice: a systematic review of rigorous evaluations. *Lancet* 1993;**342**:1317–22.

7 NHS Centre for Reviews and Dissemination. *Database of Abstracts of Reviews of Effectiveness.* York: NHS Centre for Reviews and Dissemination, 1998.

8 Oxman AD, Guyatt GH. The science of reviewing research. *Ann New York Acad Sci* 1993;**703**:125–33.

9 Oxman AD. Checklists for review articles. *BMJ* 1994;**309**:648–51.

10 Lomas J. Words without action? The production, dissemination, and impact of consensus recommendations. *Annu Rev Public Health* 1991;**12**:41–65.

11 Grilli R, Lomas J. Evaluating the message: the relationship between compliance rate and the subject of a practice guideline. *Med Care* 1994;**32**:202–13.

12 Oxman AD, Thomson MA, Davis DA, Haynes RB. No magic bullets: a systematic review of 102 trials of interventions to improve general practice. *CMAJ* 1995;**153**:1423–31.

13 Beaudry JS. The effectiveness of continuing medical education: a quantitative synthesis. *J Cont Educ Health Prof* 1989;**9**:285–307.

14 Davis DA, Thomson MA, Oxman AD, Haynes RB. Changing physician performance: A systematic review of the effect of continuing medical education strategies. *JAMA* 1995; **274**:700–5.

15 Mugford M, Banfield P, O'Hanlon M. Effects of feedback of information on clinical practice: a review. *BMJ* 1991;**303**:398–402.

16 Buntinx F, Winkens R, Grol R, Knottnerus JA. Influencing diagnostic and preventive performance in ambulatory care by feedback and reminders. A review. *Fam Prac* 1993; **10**:219–28.

17 Johnston ME, Langton KB, Haynes RB, Mathieu A. Effects of computer-based clinical decision support systems on clinician performance and patient outcome: a critical appraisal of research. *Ann Intern Med* 1994;**120**:135–42.

18 Austin SM, Balas EA, Mitchell JA, Ewigman BG. *Effect of physician reminders on preventive care: meta-analysis of randomized clinical trials.* Proc Annu Symp Comput Appl Med Care 1994; 121–4.

19 Wensing M, Grol R. Single and combined strategies for implementing changes in primary care: a literature review. *Int J Qual Health Care* 1994; **6**:115–32.

20 Waddell DL. The effects of continuing education on nursing practice: a meta-analysis. *J Cont Educ Nursing* 1991;**22**:113–18.

21 Yano EM, Fink A, Hirsch SH, Robbins AS, Rubenstein LV. Helping practices reach primary care goals. Lessons from the literature. *Arch Intern Med* 1995;**155**:1146–56.

22 Soumerai SB, McLaughlin TJ, Avorn J. Improving drug prescribing in primary care: a critical analysis of the experimental literature. *Milbank Q* 1989;**67**:268–317.

23 Lomas J, Haynes RB. A taxonomy and critical review of tested strategies for the application of clinical practice recommendations: from "official" to "individual" clinical policy. *Am J Prev Med* 1988;**4**:77–94.

24 Gyorkos TW, Tannenbaum TN, Abrahamowicz M, *et al.* Evaluation of the effectiveness of immunization delivery methods. *Can J Public Health* 1994;**85(1)**:S14–S30.

25 Mandelblatt J, Kanetsky PA. Effectiveness of interventions to enhance physician screening for breast cancer. *J Fam Pract* 1995;**40**:162–71.

26 Silagy C, Lancaster T, Gray S, Fowler G. The effectiveness of training health professionals to provide smoking cessation interventions: systematic review of randomised controlled trials. *Qual Health Care* 1995;**3**:193–8.

27 Lomas J, Anderson GM, Domnick-Pierre K, Vayda E, Enkin MW, Hannah WJ. Do practice guidelines guide practice? The effect of a consensus statement on the practise of physicians. *New Engl J Med* 1989;**321**:1306–11.

28 Whiting-O'Keefe QE, Henke C, Simborg DW. Choosing the correct unit of analysis in medical care experiements. *Med Care* 1984;**22**:1101–14.

29 Grol R. Implementing guidelines in general practice care. *Qual Health Care* 1992;**1**: 184–91.

30 Donner A, Birkett N, Buck C. Randomisation by cluster: sample size requirements and analysis. *Am J Epidemiol* 1981;**114**:906–14.

31 NHS Research and Development Programme. *Methods to promote the implementation of research findings in the NHS – priorities for evaluation.* Report to the NHS Central Research and Development Committee. Leeds: Department of Health, 1995.

32 Freemantle N, Grilli R, Grimshaw JM, Oxman A. Implementing the findings of medical research: the Cochrane Collaboration on Effective Professional Practice. *Qual Health Care* 1995;**4**:45–7.

5 Implementing research findings into practice: beyond the information deficit model

THERESA M MARTEAU, AMANDA SOWDEN, AND
DAVID ARMSTRONG

Implicit models of changing health professionals' behaviour

The belief that new knowledge changes behaviour lies at the heart of professional practice. Medical students are transformed into medical practitioners through the inculcation of knowledge; specialist training requires a further encounter with more advanced knowledge, while professional development is built around acquiring the latest knowledge through "continuing medical education". Indeed, when exploring the characteristics of professional status, Freidson identified possession of an esoteric knowledge base, alongside commitment to an altruistic ideal, as marking out a profession from other forms of occupational organisation.[1]

However, the problem with the view that providing new knowledge produces new behaviour – an information deficit model of behaviour change – is that as an explanation it lacks both empirical and theoretical support. For example, in their overview of systematic reviews of interventions to promote implementation of research findings by practitioners, Bero and colleagues noted that there was good evidence to show that passive dissemination of information, such as mailing educational materials, was ineffective (see Chapter 4). While information may be necessary for behaviour change, it is rarely sufficient, as is illustrated by the consistent finding that patients are poor at adhering to medical advice.[2]

The problems with an information deficit model have been recognised in the education field by attempts to reconceptualise learning as an active process rather than the passive assimilation of information. In this new educational model, emphasis is placed on the learner as an adult who learns by reflection,[3] by problem-solving and involvement,[4] and by self-assessment;[5] this model therefore opposes androgogy or adult learning to traditional pedagogy in which the learner is a passive recipient of information.

Nevertheless, despite their greater sophistication and plausibility, adult learning models still pose explanatory and empirical problems. On the one hand, if (adult) learning is defined in terms of behaviour change then explanation becomes rather circular; on the other hand, if "learning" and behaviour are kept separate then the relationship between the two remains unresolved. The finding that a more "active" learning experience is more likely to change behaviour than a passive one still embodies the idea that the problem is one of information transfer: all that changes is the subtlety with which it is transmitted.[6]

Given the specific problem of how to implement the results of research into practice, a number of models have emerged that try to understand the process of changing health professionals' behaviour.[7,8] These models frequently draw on the idea of "active" learning and combine this with concepts taken from descriptive work on diffusion of innovation and technology transfer in other areas. But such models neglect a long tradition within the behavioural and social sciences of understanding and explaining behaviour.[9] The purpose of this chapter is to describe some of the psychological models of behaviour that have been used and some that could be used, as the basis for designing effective interventions to change practitioners' behaviour. While sometimes used to explain and change behaviour at an organisational level, these models focus predominantly upon the level of the individual. Research using such models show that health professionals' behaviour is subject to similar influences to that of non-health professionals.[10]

The atheoretical nature of much of the research on methods of implementing results of research into practice can be illustrated by the lack of theoretical grounding in studies in this area. We randomly selected 54 studies evaluating interventions to change health professionals' behaviour from a sample of 284 titles in three areas of clinical practice – prevention, diagnosis, and treatment – from the Cochrane Collaboration on Effective Professional Practice (CCEPP) database.[11] Three types of intervention were used, with more than one being used in some studies:

(1) provision of information, in various forms, including research-based guidelines, leaflets, and educational sessions (n = 30)
(2) provision of reminders such as stickers on patients' records to prompt the clinician to perform a particular action (n = 29)
(3) the use of audit and feedback, where information about performance is provided over a period of time (n = 5).

Only two of the papers reviewed made direct reference to the choice of intervention being guided by a theory or formal body of knowledge.[12,13]

Explicit approaches to understanding and changing behaviour: psychological models

If medicine lacks a coherent theoretical model of behaviour change, perhaps the problem with psychology is that it has a surfeit! However, despite the great number of identifiable models, two broad theoretical roots – learning theory and social-cognition models – can be identified which provide different explanations for why people behave in the way that they do and therefore offer different approaches to behaviour change.

Learning theory

Behaviourism, based on learning theory, provides an explanation of how behaviour originates, is maintained, and changed. It differs from models of behaviour such as psychoanalysis in emphasising that behaviour is controlled by its environmental consequences as opposed to being the result of internalised experiences of the distant past. One of the main principles of learning theory that has informed many interventions to change behaviour is that of operant conditioning. Once known as the Law of Effect, it states that behaviour which is followed by positive consequences will tend to be repeated, whereas behaviour followed by unpleasant consequences will occur less frequently. A variety of techniques such as imitation, role play, feedback, positive reinforcement, and punishment can be used to develop, establish, or change a behaviour. The behaviourist paradigm requires an analysis of existing behaviour in order to know how to change it; this is often represented by the ABC acronym, stressing the need to understand the **a**ntecedents of a behaviour, the context in which the **b**ehaviour occurs, and its **c**onsequences. The next step of changing behaviour usually involves three tasks: establishing and maintaining a new behaviour and, where necessary, extinguishing the existing behaviour.[14]

Behavioural approaches have mainly been used in psychiatric contexts so that examples of their use in changing professionals' behaviour are few. Payment sanctions as a form of punishment for inappropriate use of injections and rehearsal of communication skills are two instances where a behavioural approach has been effective at changing health professionals' behaviour.[15,16] Other interventions that address consequences, such as fee-for-service, target payments, and clinical audit, might be seen to have their effects through operant conditioning.

The main criticism of behavioural approaches has been that they treat human behaviour like a Pavlovian dog – get the cues right and change will result. But people are different in that they give meaning to their situations so that a financial reward for one practitioner can seem like an immoral bribe to another. The importance of these individual meanings has been addressed over the last 25 years with the integration of cognitive factors into behavioural approaches to changing behaviour, mainly in psychiatric contexts.[17] This is reflected in the expanded ABC analysis to be AA'BC where A' denotes emotions and cognitions, thus recognising that it is the perception of events not events *per se* that drive behaviour.

Nevertheless, the current shift away from a view of behaviour as primarily determined by the environment towards one that involves cognition and individual choice has meant that the behavioural tradition has been relatively neglected by psychologists working in general medical contexts. In doing so, we have perhaps ignored one of the most powerful models of behaviour change.

Social cognition models

These models share a basic premise that it is how people think about a situation, a threat, or a behaviour that determines what they do. They differ in the factors they identify as most important in predicting behaviour. Some of these models have been developed to explain behaviour outside of the health context, such as the theory of reasoned action, while others have been developed specifically to explain health related behaviour of patients, such as the health belief model.[18,19] Three sets of beliefs that have emerged as important in determining behaviour are:

1 perceived benefits weighed against perceived barriers to the action[20]
2 perceptions of the attitudes of important others to the behaviour[18]
3 self-efficacy, or belief in one's ability to perform a behaviour.[21,22]

Put more simply, before changing their behaviour, an individual is likely to ask: is this worthwhile, what do others think about it, and can I do it?

A further refinement of these models is the incorporation of an individual's readiness for change as a predictor of the likelihood of behaviour change.[23,24] These stages-of-change models see behaviour change as a process and whether someone changes their behaviour depends on where they are in terms of awareness of a threat and motivation and ability to behave to reduce the threat. While such models seem intuitively appealing, evidence that people proceed in a timely fashion along a continuum from awareness to change is currently lacking.[25,26]

The test of the usefulness of all these models is in their ability to inform the design of effective interventions.[27] While these models have been used in tens of thousands of studies to predict behaviour, there have been very few studies in which researchers have attempted to change behaviour by altering cognitions that are predictive of behaviour.[28] While some of these have successfully altered cognitions and thereby behaviour,[29,30] others have found that changing beliefs that predict behaviour does not lead to behaviour change.[31]

Merging the strengths of both behavioural and social cognition models, as has happened in cognitive behaviour therapy, may prove a more effective way of changing behaviour, including that of health professionals.[17] Such a development requires conceptual as well as empirically based work.

Integrating implicit and explicit models of behaviour change

The value of psychological models in changing health professionals' behaviour needs to be seen in the wider context of the relationship between researcher and researched. Those who are developing strategies to promote the uptake of the research findings might hold an explicit model of behaviour change (some of which have been described above), but the clinicians whose behaviour is to be changed have their own ideas about whether and how such change might be effected. This means that behaviour change is not a one-sided business, a case of an enlightened intervention trying to change an old-fashioned clinician, but a process of negotiating whose model will prevail and whose behaviour will be changed. For example, those attempting to promote the uptake of research findings might dismiss the clinician's clinical experience as outmoded; equally, the clinicians might reject the applicability of the so-called evidence to their own work. Indeed, the clinician, through resistance, may succeed in changing some of the beliefs, and possibly behaviour, of those promoting uptake of research findings. In short, a failed intervention from the point of view of the persons trying to change a clinician's behaviour may be a successful one from the clinician's perspective! In other words, the interpretations that professionals place on their own behaviours, such as the information deficit model, might be "mistaken" but are themselves factors that need addressing if interventions are to succeed. For example, professionals who believe that their behaviour changes in response to new knowledge may be resistant to being involved in a system based overtly on rewards and punishment.

And of course, these caveats might apply to writers as well as to investigators! The mere writing of this chapter, and indeed the existence of medical journals, can be seen as subscribing to an information deficit model of human behaviour. Information, of course, has functions other than changing behaviour, such as to increase understanding, to amuse, and to give power. As we have argued, on its own, information transfer is unlikely to change the behaviour of the reader but perhaps, if it is coupled with an understanding of how information functions as an antecedent to behaviour and informing cognitions about how behaviour is changed, it may work more effectively.

Acknowledgement

Theresa M Marteau is funded by The Wellcome Trust.

References

1 Freidson E. *Profession of medicine: a study of the sociology of applied knowledge.* New York: Dodd Mead, 1970.
2 Miechenbaum D, Turk DC. *Facilitating treatment adherence: a practitioner's guidebook.* New York and London: Plenum Press, 1987.
3 Schon DA. *The reflective practitioner.* New York: Basic Books, 1983.
4 Knowles R. *The adult learner: a neglected species.* Houston: Gulf, 1977.
5 Coles C. Self-assessment and medical audit: an educational appraisal. *BMJ* 1989;**299**: 807–8.
6 Davies DA, Thomson MA, Oxman AD, Haynes RB. Changing physician performance: a systematic review of the effect of continuing medical education strategies. *JAMA* 1995; **274**:700–5.
7 Haines A, Jones R. Implementing findings of research. *BMJ* 1994;**308**:1488–92.
8 Kitson A, Ahmed LB, Harvey G, Seers K, Thompson DR. From research to practice: one organizational model for promoting research-based practice. *J Advanced Nursing* 1996; **23**:430–40.
9 Dawson S. Never mind solutions: what are the issues? Lessons of industrial technology transfer for quality in health care. *Qual Health Care* 1995;**4**:197–203.
10 Marteau TM, Johnston M. Health professionals: a source of variance in health outcomes. *Psychology and Health* 1990;**5**:47–58.
11 Bero L, Freemantle N, Grilli R, Grimshaw JM, Harvey E, Oxman AD. ed. *The Cochrane Collaboration on Effective Professional Practice Module of the Cochrane Database of Systematic Reviews.* 3rd edn. London: BMJ Publishing Group, 1996.
12 Wing Hong S, Ching TY, Fung JPM, Seto WL. The employment of ward opinion leaders for continuing education in the hospitals. *Med Teach* 1990;**12**:209–17.
13 Brown LF, Keily PA, Spencer AJ. Evaluation of a continuing education intervention: "periodontics in general practice". *Comm Dent Oral Epidemiol* 1994;**22**:441–7.
14 Kanfer FH, Goldstein AP. ed. *Helping people change: a textbook of methods.* New York: Pergamon Press, 1975.
15 Brook RH, Williams KN. Effect of medical care on the use of injections: a study of the New Mexico experimental medical care review organization. *Ann Intern Med* 1976;**515**: 509–15.
16 Kottke TE, Brekke ML, Solberg LI, Hughes JR. A randomized trial to increase smoking intervention by physicians: doctors helping smokers, round 1. *JAMA* 1989;**261**:2101–6.
17 Hawton K, Salkovskis PM, Kirk J, Clark DM. ed. *Cognitive behaviour therapy for psychiatric problems: a practical guide.* Oxford: Oxford University Press, 1992.
18 Fishbein M, Ajzen I. *Belief, attitude, intention, and behavior.* New York: Wiley, 1975.
19 Becker MH. The health belief model and sick role behavior. *Health Education Monographs* 1974;**2**:409,419.

41

20 Janz NK, Becker MH. The health belief model: a decade later. *Health Educ Q* 1984;**11**: 1–47.
21 Bandura A. *Social foundations of thought and action: a cognitive social theory.* Englewood Cliffs, NJ: Prentice-Hall, 1986.
22 Schwartzer R. Self-efficacy in the adoption and maintenance of health behaviours: theoretical approaches and a new model. In: Schwartzer R. ed. *Self-efficacy: thought control of action.* Washington: Hemisphere Publishing Corporation, 1992.
23 Prochaska JO, DiClemente CC. *The transtheoretical approach: crossing traditional boundaries of therapy.* Homewood, IL: Dow Jones Irwin, 1984.
24 Weinstein ND. The precaution adoption process. *Health Psychol* 1988;**7**:355–86.
25 Sutton S. The past predicts the future: interpreting behaviour – behaviour relationships in social psychological models of health behaviours. In: Rutter DR, Quine L. eds. *Social psychology and health: European perspectives.* Aldershot and Vermont: Avebury, 1994.
26 Ashworth P. Breakthrough or bandwagon? Are interventions tailored to Stage of Change more effective than non-staged interventions? *Health Educ J* 1997;**56**:166–74.
27 Fishbein M. Foreword. In: Terry DJ, Gallois C, McCamish M. *The theory of reasoned action: its application to AIDS-related behaviour.* Oxford: Pergamon Press, 1993.
28 Conner M, Norman P. Health behaviour. In: Johnston M, Johnston D. ed. *Health psychology. Comprehensive clinical psychology, vol 7.* Oxford: Elsevier Science Ltd. In press.
29 Maibach E, Flora JA, Nass C. Changes in self-efficacy and health behavior in response to a minimal community health campaign. *Health Comm* 1991;**3**:1–15.
30 Wurtele SK, Maddux JE. Relative contributions of protection motivation components in predicting exercise intentions and behaviour. *Health Psychol* 1987;**6**:453–66.
31 Weinstein ND, Sandman PM, Roberts NE. Perceived susceptibility and self-protective behaviour: a field experiment to encourage home radon testing. *Health Psychol* 1991;**10**: 25–33.

6 Roles for lay people in the implementation of healthcare research

SANDY OLIVER, VIKKI ENTWISTLE, AND
ELLEN HODNETT

Introduction

As patients or potential patients, lay people as well as professionals have a
vested interest in ensuring the availability and appropriate use of health
care interventions which rigorous evaluations have shown to be effective.
However, uninformed or misinformed patients, consumer groups, and wider
publics can hinder the implementation of research findings. Recognition
of this has fuelled enthusiasm for the provision of research-based
information about health care effectiveness to lay audiences alongside the
encouragement of greater lay involvement in health care decision making.
It is hoped that informed consumers will expect and demand effective
forms of care.

The provision of good quality information to all those involved in health
care decisions is extremely important but often not sufficient to overcome
the various professional, financial, practical, and social barriers to research
implementation. In this chapter, we consider some of the ways in which
lay people might help to identify and overcome these barriers and hence
contribute to attempts to base health care policy and practice on sound
research findings. After a brief consideration of the policy context and
conceptual issues, we use selected examples, particularly of British and
Canadian initiatives, to illustrate ways in which patients, consumer groups,
and others might be encouraged and enabled to facilitate beneficial changes
in health care. We also consider how approaches to lay involvement might
be evaluated.

Policy context and conceptual issues

The implementation of research findings is explicitly encouraged with the movement towards evidence based health care[1] and policies promoting clinical effectiveness.[2] It is also encouraged by many of those advocating greater patient involvement in decisions about individual health care and greater lay input into decisions about health care policy and practice.[3] Research evidence can be interpreted and used in a variety of ways: some evidence of effectiveness does not convince those who judge care by a broad range of functional and psychosocial outcomes.[4] Furthermore, opinions vary about the role which personal or social preference should play in health care decisions. People who place differing emphases on research evidence and personal preference may hold a variety of possibly conflicting views about the aims of research implementation, the appropriateness of different approaches to it, the roles which patients, consumer advocates, and other lay groups can usefully play, and the criteria by which implementation initiatives should be judged. The consistent delivery of a particular form of care to all people with a given condition and circumstance, for example, could be seen as an indicator of a highly successful implementation of an effective form of care or of limited opportunities for individual patients to exercise their own choices.

What roles might lay people play?

Lay involvement in research implementation activities is encouraged because it is believed to add value to those activities and/or because it is seen as politically appropriate. Lay people with diverse backgrounds and experiences might contribute to aspects of research implementation in a range of ways. Policy makers, managers, and practitioners who are trying to encourage research implementation might find it helpful to consider three related questions.

1   Who might bring what insights, skills, and other attributes?

Individual patients and their carers have particular insights based on their experiences of illness and of particular health services, and may have a strong personal interest in the implementation of specific research findings. Condition-specific consumer organisations which facilitate contact between patients, offer information, advice, or services, and campaign on behalf of their constituent group can often present the diverse views of their members. Generic consumer organisations working in the health sector, and umbrella

44

organisations of patient groups, can ensure that patient perspectives are kept on the agenda and that consumerist principles are not neglected.

2 To what aspects of the implementation process might they contribute?

Lay perspectives might usefully inform, and lay efforts facilitate:

- the prioritisation of research messages for implementation
- target setting
- the selection and execution of activities to promote implementation
- the evaluation of initiatives.

If, as seems plausible, the perceived relevance of research affects its implementation, then lay involvement in research prioritisation and design may also enhance the research implementation effort.

3 How will their contribution best be encouraged and facilitated?

Even if it is not their primary intention, lay people may influence the implementation of research in a variety of ways both while discussing their own care with health professionals and by contributing to decisions about health care policy and practice. A few illustrative examples are provided below.

Individual patients in consultations

Interactions between health professionals and patients take many forms, and there are several models describing the different roles which may be played by each in deciding which forms of health care will be given.[5] Clearly, there is potential for both health professionals and patients to influence the extent to which health care reflects research evidence of effectiveness. Interventions to influence health professionals' knowledge, attitudes, and behaviour have been discussed in other chapters. We focus here on interventions designed to influence patients' contributions.

Various information-giving interventions have been developed which aim either to persuade people to accept a particular treatment option or to help them make an informed choice between options. Opinions about the appropriateness of the two approaches will vary according to the types of decisions and the nature of the options being considered, and with views about the relative importance of research evidence and individual choice.

45

The health care systems within which decisions are made are also important as they vary with the scope they can afford for individual preferences.[6]

The persuasive information-giving approach has been used with some success in attempts to fully implement immunisation programmes[7] and to encourage uptake of preventive health care services among adult populations.[8] It can also be seen in efforts to encourage acceptance of generic rather than brand name prescribing. Reminders for patients and other attempts to improve adherence to effective medication regimes may also be viewed as attempts to implement research evidence.

The provision of information which explicitly outlines and offers choices between different forms of care is most commonly seen where health professionals recognise there are trade-offs to be made between the benefits and risks of different options. In the UK, the Informed Choice initiative aims both to encourage research-based practice and to help women make informed choices about maternity care. Pairs of leaflets for women and health professionals summarise the best available research evidence about the effectiveness of interventions such as routine ultrasound in early pregnancy, fetal monitoring, and social support during labour.[9]

Interactive media have also been used to permit patients to explore a range of options and to proceed through them at their own pace. For example, the Foundation for Informed Decision Making in the United States has developed a range of interactive videos and supporting written materials for patients.[10] The interactive video system is being evaluated in the US and UK for benign prostatic hypertrophy and, more recently, hormone replacement therapy and preliminary studies show that it is well received by patients.[11,12] Although expensive to develop, sophisticated multimedia systems may ultimately prove to be cost-effective.[13] It has been suggested that in considering shared decision making, the issue of problem solving should be separated from decision making. The former involves identifying the single best solution to the problem and the latter involves selecting the most desired bundle of outcomes. A study using these concepts in patients undergoing angiography showed that patients overwhelmingly wanted the problem-solving tasks, which required technical expertise, to be performed by or with the clinician, but wanted to be actively involved in the selection of appropriate outcomes.[14] Preference for handing control to clinicians was greater for vignettes which involved life-threatening problems than for those which involved mainly morbidity or quality of life. A recent review article has discussed the growing but still sparse literature on shared decision making and made the case for more high quality research in this area.[15]

Patients may have access to various information sources, not all of which will reflect the available research evidence. They may need help to appraise and interpret what information they have.

In addition to intervening with the provision of information, attempts have been made to encourage people to ask about the effectiveness of treatments which their health professionals suggest and to enquire about alternatives. Several studies suggest that training and role-modelling techniques can help patients to ask more questions and elicit information more effectively during consultations.[16-18] The extent to which such interventions increase the likelihood of treatment decisions reflecting available research is less clear.

Lay contributions to decisions about health care policy and practice

Lay representatives serving on a range of policy and management committees or project teams may find themselves in a position to influence the implementation of research. Most obviously, there has been increasing interest in recent years in lay involvement in health care audit activities and in the development and use of clinical practice guidelines, although practice in both areas has tended to fall short of stated ideals. Lay involvement in audit is officially endorsed in the UK but it is not yet widespread and lay contributions have, for various reasons, tended to be limited,[19] with many initiatives comprising little more than user satisfaction surveys.[20] Similarly, lay involvement in guideline development has been patchy and of uncertain impact.[21,22]

Patients and consumer advocates have played significant roles in implementation projects. Several of the ideas, examples, and recommendations presented in this chapter were identified during a workshop convened by the NHS Research and Development Programme in which consumer representatives explored the potential roles of health service users in research implementation and helped set the agenda in this area (see Box 6.1).[23]

Lay contributions are increasingly seen in the development of information materials. In the UK, for example, women from various backgrounds with dysfunctional uterine bleeding contributed to a multifaceted strategy to promote effective management of the condition by helping to develop leaflets to encourage women to seek appropriate professional help.[24] Focus groups of patients also influenced the content and presentation of a research-based leaflet to facilitate informed decisions about the treatment of cataract.[25] In Canada, the lay member of the Maternity Care Guideline Implementation Demonstration Project in Ontario played an active role in all aspects of the design and implementation of the project, and was responsible for the development of the strategies and materials needed to educate the public about effective and ineffective forms of care.[26] People with a genuine experience of the patient's perspective can be vital in helping

47

Box 6.1   Questions to ask when embarking on research implementation (identified by lay representatives)

Who will define the problems and goals?

Who will initiate, manage and fund projects?

Will all stakeholders be involved from the beginning?

At what stage(s) in the process will service users be involved?

Will specific roles for service users be identified?

Which lay people will be involved? How will they be identified and chosen?

Will they be able to express the views of other lay people?

What skills do lay people already have, and what will they need to develop?

Who will set quality standards for monitoring the implementation?

What resources will be available to support lay involvement?

How stressful will the implementation process be for everyone involved?

Will the implementation strategy achieve desirable and lasting change?

Will everyone involved consider the achievements worthwhile?

Will purchasers' contracts subsequently include criteria chosen by lay people?

Will the experience of involving lay people be recorded and reflected upon for the benefit of subsequent exercises?

Will professionals appreciate the contributions made by lay people and look forward to working with them or their peers again?

identify information needs and to ensure that information is presented in an understandable, acceptable, and useful way.

Successful partnerships in implementation activities are likely to require early and continuing involvement of people who can speak from the perspective of health service users and are well informed about technical issues.[22,27] The challenges of multidisciplinary working are increased when teams include people who have not been trained as health professionals, as Grimshaw and colleagues observed in the case of guideline development:

> . . . inherent professional hierarchies . . . and mutual ignorance of different professionals' skills and *modus operandi* mean that skilled leadership and adequate time are required to ensure that all panel members are actively involved in guideline development. These issues become more important when patients are involved in guideline development groups: the asymmetry of information, the perceived status of health care professionals, and the technical discussions involved in guideline development make it difficult for patients to contribute actively. . . .[28]

Practical, technical, and moral support may be required if the contribution of lay representatives is to be maximised. Training schemes have already been developed for the purpose of overcoming some of the barriers faced by lay people trying to participate in activities led by professionals. The Critical Appraisal Skills Programme (CASP) has offered technical training in the interpretation of research reports to consumer health information providers[29] and members of Maternity Service Liaison committees (multidisciplinary groups for discussing and making recommendations about local services). The Voices project has provided background information about health services management and training in committee procedures and assertiveness to lay committee members.[30] A newly commissioned Centre for Health Information Quality will work with a range of information producers and providers to improve the National Health Service's capacity to provide high quality information for patients and the wider public about treatment options and outcomes.[31] Among other things, it will encourage critical reading of information about health care.

Lay influences on policy and practice are not always contained within health service or professionally led contexts. Specific interest groups sometimes feel that they must take the initiative themselves. For example, the (UK) National Childbirth Trust has developed its own policy statement about the generation and use of research evidence.[27] Some groups engage in active campaigning activities, either for or (perhaps misguidedly) against practices which represent the implementation of research, sometimes in open conflict with health professional groups.

The lay media may play an important role in such campaigning activities and more generally in promoting or hindering the uptake of research messages. For example, media coverage which drew attention to high hysterectomy rates in the Swiss canton of Ticino was apparently followed by a drop in rates,[32] although the extent to which the media cause change, as opposed to reflecting it, is not clear.

Evaluation

The effects of different approaches to lay involvement in implementation activities are to a large extent unknown. Ideally, lay involvement in implementation needs to culminate in lay involvement in its evaluation. For instance, Portuguese women have helped to design and implement methods of inviting the underscreened in Toronto, Canada, to have Pap Smears[33] and are now members of the trial-steering committee evaluating the intervention.

With so much potential for lay involvement to enhance research implementation, we are likely to see more innovative initiatives in the near future. Participatory principles should be matched by clear descriptions and evaluations of processes, rigorous outcome evaluations, and critical discussions of successful and unsuccessful initiatives. Developmental work should be accompanied by good evaluative research which draws on professional and lay perspectives from the outset.

Acknowledgements

We would like to thank all those who participated in the workshop held in November 1994 to inform the Central R&D Committee Advisory Group on the Implementation of Research Findings: Bola Arowinde, Jane Bradburn, Alison Clarke, Hafize Ece, Tina Funnell, Hilary Gilbert, Gill Gyte, Christabel Hilliard, Deborah Khudabux, Tara Lamont, Jo Marsden, Becky Miles, Carole Myer, Belinda Pratton, Ann Smith, Monika Temple, Hazel Thornton, Peter Willis.

Some of the ideas incorporated in this paper have been discussed with Amanda Sowden, Ian Watt, and Trevor Sheldon.

Ann Oakley and Barbara Stocking provided helpful comments on a draft of the text.

References

1 Sackett DL, Rosenburg WMC, Gray JAM, Haynes RB, Richardson WS. Evidence based medicine: what it is and what it isn't. *BMJ* 1995;**312**:71–2.
2 NHS Executive. *Promoting Clinical Effectiveness: a framework for action in and through the NHS*. Leeds: NHS Executive, 1996.
3 Hope T. *Evidence based patient choice*. London: Kings Fund, 1996.
4 Oliver S. Exploring lay perspectives on questions of effectiveness. In: Maynard A, Chalmers I. eds. *Non-random reflections on health services research*. London: BMJ Publishing Group, 1997.
5 Charles C, Gafni A, Whelan T. Shared decision making in the medical encounter: what does it mean? (Or it takes at least two to tango). *Soc Sci Med* 1997;**44**:681–92.
6 Royce RG. Observations on the NHS internal market: will the dodo get the last laugh? *BMJ* 1995;**311**:431–3.
7 Hodnett ED. Support from caregivers for socially disadvantaged mothers. In: Enkin MW, Keirse MJNC, Renfrew MJ, Neilson JP. ed. *Pregnancy and Childbirth Module of The Cochrane Database of Systematic Reviews* [updated 6 September 1996]. Available in The Cochrane Library [database on disk and CD-ROM]; The Cochrane Collaboration, Issue 3; Oxford: Update Software, 1996. Updated quarterly. Available from: BMJ Publishing Group, London.
8 Dickey LL. Promoting preventative care with patient-held mini-records: a review. *Patient Education and Counselling* 1993;**20**:37–47.
9 Anderson T. Using evidence to empower childbearing women. *Midwives* 1996;**1296**:12–14.
10 Kasper JF, Mullew AG, Wennberg JE. Developing shared decision making programs to improve the quality of health care. *Qual Rev Bull* 1992;**18**:182–90.
11 Barry MJ, Fowler FJ, Mulley AG, Henderson JV, Wennberg JE. Patient reactions to a program designed to facilitate patient participation in treatment decisions for benign prostatic hyperplasia. *Med Care* 1995;**33**:771–82.
12 Shepperd S, Coulter A, Farmer A. Using interactive videos in general practice to inform patients about treatment choices: a pilot study. *Fam Pract* 1995;**12**:443–7.

13 Nease RF, Owens DK. A method for estimating the cost-effectiveness of incorporation of patient preferences into practical guidelines. *Medical Decision Making* 1994;**14**:382–92.
14 Deber RB, Kraetschmer N, Irvine J. What role do patients wish to play in treatment decision making? *Arch Intern Med* 1996;**156**:1414–20.
15 Coulter A. Partnerships with patients: the pros and cons of shared clinical decision making. *J Health Serv Res Policy* 1997;**2**:112–20.
16 Anderson LA, DeVellis BM, DeVellis RF. Effects of modelling on patient communication, satisfaction and knowledge. *Med Care* 1987;**25**:1044–56.
17 Butow PN, Dunn SM, Tattershall MHN, Jones QJ. Patient participation in the cancer consultation: evaluation of a question prompt sheet. *Ann Oncol* 1994;**5**:199–204.
18 Frederikson LG, Bull PE. Evaluation of a patient education leaflet designed to improve communication in medical consultations. *Patient Education and Counselling* 1995;**25**:51–7.
19 Kelson M. *Consumer involvement initiatives in clinical audit and outcomes: a review of developments and issues in the identifications of good practice*. London: College of Health, 1995.
20 Kelson M, Redpath L. Promoting user involvement in clinical audit: surveys of audit committees in primary and secondary care. *J Clin Effect* 1996;**1**:14–18.
21 Bastian H. Raising the standard: practice guidelines and consumer participation. *Int J Qual Health Care* 1996;**8**:485–90.
22 Duff LA, Kelson M, Marriott S, McIntosh A, *et al*. Clinical guidelines; involving patients and users of services. *J Clin Effect* 1996;**1**:104–12.
23 Oliver S. *Involving health service users in the implementation of research findings*. A report to the CRDC Advisory Group on Research Implementation, 1995.
24 Dunning M, McQuay H, Milne R. Getting a grip. *Health Services Journal* 1994;**April**: 24–5.
25 Entwistle VA, Watt IS, Davis H, Dickson R, Pickard DA, Rosser J. Developing information materials to present the findings of technology assessment to consumers: the experience of the NHS Centre for Reviews and Dissemination. *Int J Tech Assess Health Care* 1998; **14**. In press.
26 Anderson G, The MCGIDP Group. Maternity Care Guideline Implementation Demonstration Project. Ontario, Canada: Medical Research Council of Canada. In progress.
27 Oliver S. How can health service users contribute to the NHS research and development programme? *BMJ* 1995;**310**:1318–20.
28 Grimshaw J, Eccles M, Russell I. Developing clinically valid practice guidelines. *J Eval Clin Pract* 1995;**1**(1):37–48.
29 Milne R, Oliver S. Evidence based consumer health information: developing teaching in critical appraisal skills. *Int J Qual Health Care* 1996;**8**(5):439–45.
30 Training and support for maternity user representatives. *New Generation* 1995;**14**(4):22.
31 Department of Health. Primary care: delivering the future. London: The Stationery Office, 1996.
32 Domenighetti G, Luraschi P, Casabianca A, Gutzwiller F, Spinelli A, Pedrinis E. Effect of information campaigns by the mass media on hysterectomy rates. *Lancet* 1988;**332**: 1470–3.
33 Rael E, Miller A, Hodnett E, *et al*. *Development and evaluation of invitations for Portugese-speaking women to have Pap tests*. PhD thesis. Toronto, Canada: University of Toronto. In progress.

7 Implementing research findings in clinical practice

ANNA DONALD AND RUAIRIDH MILNE

People must be able to learn and implement new knowledge if they are to adapt to change. Yet it is still remarkably difficult for doctors and nurses in the National Health Service to sift through the thousands of new research findings appearing in the literature and use the relatively few robust findings relevant to their own practice. Current educational methods, from undergraduate training to continuing medical education courses, still rely predominantly upon non-problem-based teaching methods, such as didactic lectures, which do not teach skills for accessing new knowledge. Moreover, the need to integrate research findings into clinical practice is rarely recognised in the provision of ward computing facilities, regional and national library services, nor the investment decisions of Trusts or primary care centres.

What alternatives exist? How may we better proceed in future? In this chapter we examine how one hospital firm attempted to implement research findings into practice. We draw from medical and anthropological literature, as well as a "collective" case study derived from our experience of training clinicians to evaluate and use evidence over the past three years in London and Oxford, confirmed recently by others' experiences in North America, The Netherlands, and Australia.

Case study: Dr Franks' firm

Dr Franks runs a busy medical firm in a London district general hospital. Until recently, Dr Franks and his team made most medical decisions based on previous experience and a modest sprinkling of "the literature". Altogether, he and his team read three medical journals – the *British Medical Journal*, *The Lancet*, and *New England Journal of Medicine* – for approximately three hours each week (half an hour each for Dr Franks, his senior registrar, and registrar, and 45 minutes each for the two senior house officers). The two house officers did not have time to read anything. While respectable, the journals did not provide them with good "quality filters" of the thousands of articles published each month. No firm member had been trained to evaluate published evidence assessing patient care, so they could not apply a rigorous quality filter themselves nor be confident of their response when presented with conflicting evidence in the recommendations of peers, drug representatives, and conference proceedings. Dr Franks' senior registrar had vaguely heard mention of databases such as the Cochrane Library and Best Evidence* that might have provided effective quality filters for information, but the ward computer was old and could scarcely run the Windows programme loaded onto it, let alone a large database on CD-ROM.

Furthermore, Dr Franks' hospital library and services left much to be desired. The local library holdings were small and frequently missing, the opening hours short, and the librarian friendly but overworked and not trained in searching efficiently for high quality information. MEDLINE back to 1986 was available on two terminals in the library but, due to vandalism, the machines themselves were locked inside a cabinet making it impossible to download information onto a floppy disk. There were no other databases available of relevance to Dr Franks' team and, even if there were, obtaining the full text article involved an inter-library loan that took at least four days and usually a week or more by the time the librarian had retrieved it from the British Library and sent it via internal mail to the ward. Also, as the library was a good ten-minute walk from the ward, neither Dr Franks nor his staff made regular use of it nor knew the librarian well enough to know what she might be able to do to improve article retrieval for the firm.

In short, with a case-load in excess of 40 patients at a time, busy takes, and virtually no support for using research findings other than using a slow and rather haphazard kind of osmosis, Dr Franks' team was unlikely to do much to upgrade its decision making capacity.

Then, during the summer, Dr Franks was approached by the research and development arm of his regional office to join a project in which team members would receive the equipment and training necessary to "find, appraise, and act on evidence":[1] a new computer (supplied by the Trust), a CD-ROM tower that could permanently store and run CD-ROMs without risking theft, three databases applicable to general medicine – the Cochrane Library (The Cochrane Collaboration, Issue 1; Oxford: Update Software, 1997, updated quarterly), MEDLINE back to 1992, and the ACP Journal Club – and basic training in critical appraisal (or literature

---

* In North America, the collection of quality-filtered abstracts produced under the title of "Best Evidence" derive from the bi-monthly supplement to the *Annals of Internal Medicine*, called the *ACP Journal Club*. A journal in its own right, it is now published also in Europe as *Evidence based Medicine* (BMJ Publications, London).

evaluation) skills from a local trainer (a public health doctor). The team decided to take part in the project. This is what happened.

First, Dr Franks decided to find out more about using research findings or "evidence" effectively in order for him to present the idea to his firm and to other people whose support he would need, including the computer staff, the Trust Executive, and the librarian. Therefore, Dr Franks asked the librarian to obtain some key self-help materials referenced in *The ScHARR guide to evidence based practice*[2] and enrolled himself on one of the "evidence based medicine" courses being held regularly in London and Oxford. Next, Dr Franks began a strategy to have everyone in the team use evidence effectively on a regular basis.

First, he explained to his team at a firm meeting how regular research appraisal or "evidence based practice" could be of value to them, and asked who might be interested in attending the training sessions in literature searching and appraisal skills. With those interested (all the doctors, one manager, two senior nurses, and one physiotherapist), Dr Franks wrote a short contract committing all parties to a minimum attendance at training sessions and to fulfilment of ward round-based "educational prescriptions" to search and appraise literature at least once a month.

Second, with the allocated regional trainer for the firm, and bearing in mind the firm's schedule of clinics and takes, Dr Franks scheduled four lunch-time and afternoon training sessions, each two hours long. However, without a locum for each session, he recognised that not all junior staff would be able to attend every training session. Also, the four sessions were not ideal for the trainer who would have preferred that the training take place intensively over a whole or two half days. However, without money to hire locums the prolonged lunch-time arrangement was the best available option.

Third, Dr Franks' team negotiated the content of the training with the regional trainer. Together, they decided to spend the first two-hour session introducing the concept of evidence based practice to the firm and teaching staff to ask specific, "searchable" questions in the literature, the second on finding the best available information in the shortest possible time, the third on appraising the information they found, and the fourth on acting on (or implementing) their appraised findings to real clinical problems[3]. Given the firm's ongoing interest in stroke management, the team trainer decided that in the third session he would ask the team to critically appraise a systematic review on stroke management from the Cochrane Library,[4] using the critical appraisal criteria outline shown in Box 7.1. In this way the training sessions were of real rather than abstract interest to the firm (i.e. they were "problem-based"), and the trainer could concurrently teach the firm the usefulness of systematic reviews and the Cochrane Library as good starting places for efficient problem solving.

54

Box 7.1 Critical appraisal criteria for review articles[5]

- Did the overview address a clearly focused question?
- Were appropriate criteria used to select articles for inclusion?
- Is it unlikely that important, relevant studies were missed?
- Was the validity of the included studies assessed?
- Were assessments of studies reproducible?
- Were the results similar from study to study?
- What are the overall results of the review?
- How precise were the results?
- Can the results be applied to my patients?
- Were all clinically important outcomes considered?

Fourth, the local librarian helped Dr Franks to install the Trust-pledged computer and CD-ROM tower, and discussed ways of speeding up the process of obtaining hard copies of articles identified on MEDLINE. For the time being, these included the installation of a plain-paper fax machine on the ward with which to fax requests (indicating the urgency of the article) and receive articles. Both acknowledged, however, that the rate-limiting step was the two to three days it took the loaning library to find, copy, and send back the article, which would require major changes to nationwide library services to alter. Hence, for the time being, the firm would rely mostly on the detailed, structured abstracts from the ACP Journal Club database which usually contained all the information needed for making a clinical decision, as well as the shorter abstracts on MEDLINE and the occasional full-text systematic review from the Cochrane Library. The ACP Journal Club abstracts and Cochrane Library reviews were particularly useful as their authors had already appraised and summarised the original articles, thus much reducing the work of the doctors.

Finally, the team decided to locate the computer and CD-ROM tower in the doctors' room where it would be both secure and accessible given doctors' unpredictable but real "downtime" between bleeps and long stretches of work.

Unfortunately, Dr Franks did not discuss the project in depth with the Trust Executive before agreeing to participate, and the promised computer arrived with only a small amount of memory, making the large databases too slow for rapid use by busy medical staff. An extra 16 RAM had to be ordered (costing £150). While the Cochrane Library looked promising, it came without detailed instructions. Therefore, Dr Franks did not realise for weeks that in addition to over 200 completed systematic reviews, it also contained a bank of 140 000 references of randomised controlled trials relevant to different clinical topics, the NHS Centre for Reviews and

Dissemination's entire Database of Abstracts of Reviews of Effectiveness (DARE), as well as articles about using evidence and contact numbers for members of the Cochrane Collaboration (Box 7.2).

Box 7.2 Information available in the 1998 volume 1 edition of The Cochrane Library (The Cochrane Collaboration, Oxford: Update Software, 1998, updated quarterly)

- The Cochrane Database of Systematic Reviews (358 entries)
  - Completed and in-progress full text of systematic reviews, pulling together results from hundreds of individual randomised controlled trials
- Database of Abstracts of Reviews of Effectiveness (1626 entries)
  - Completed and in-progress abstracts of systematic reviews, appraising results of hundreds of individual trials of different kinds
- Cochrane Controlled Trials Register (112 308 entries)
  - References for thousands of individual randomised controlled trials, each of which has reached minimal critical appraisal criteria
- Cochrane Review Methodology Database (398 entries)
  - References of articles *about* evaluating the literature, including self-help articles
- Information about the Cochrane Collaboration (84 entries)
  - Details of Cochrane Review Groups and Cochrane Collaboration contacts

---

Despite these delays, training proceeded as planned. Five months after joining the project, Dr Franks and his team are still using the skills they learnt during the afternoon training sessions, which they found good but rather sporadic and therefore much enhanced by Dr Franks' newly acquired skills that enabled him to reinforce and clarify concepts on a daily basis. Dr Frank's training role has proved crucial given the rapid turnover of junior staff and hence the ongoing need for ward-based training. In fact, the firm is getting a reputation among junior staff as a good place to train as the critical appraisal skills enable them to evaluate the literature quickly and accurately, helping them to pass membership exams.

The team has decided to restructure the firm's fortnightly journal club. Rather than present papers based on a loose discussion of their contents, staff now: (1) ask questions they are interested in answering, specifying patients, outcomes, and interventions of interest, (2) find papers using structured search strategies, and (3) evaluate what they find according to "critical appraisal" or evaluation criteria available for virtually all types of medical literature they are likely to encounter.[6]

Obtaining full texts of articles is still a real problem. However, the biggest threat to the project is that the region cannot continue to fund the subscriptions to the databases indefinitely. Without a long-term information strategy, the Trust has not yet committed to funding them, although the total cost is small, relative to the cost of defending one court suit or buying drugs for a few chronically ill patients. Dr Franks is beginning to wish that he had implemented an evaluation process earlier, so as to have some hard results to show the Trust Executive. However, with his enhanced reputation as a clinical trainer and the noise that his staff are making around the hospital about the project, he is hopeful that the Trust will continue to fund the databases and maintain the ward computer.

Discussion

Dr Franks' experience suggests that simple "diffusion" of information, whereby primary or secondary sources of research are given to clinicians without analytical and operational frameworks in which to use them, is inadequate to ensure its effective use in patient care. Rather, our and others' experience with teams like Dr Franks' strongly underscore Lomas' thesis[7] that effective implementation of research knowledge requires a restructuring of the local clinical environment and hence coordination of many people and resources both within and outside of the firm.

In his coordinated implementation model (Figure 7.1), Lomas identifies three main elements necessary for the successful implementation of knowledge into practice:

(1) the research findings packaged in a digestible form, such as the Cochrane Library, Best Evidence, and the European-based *Journal of Evidence based Medicine* that provide quality filters for hundreds of primary journals

(2) a credible dissemination body containing influential and/or authoritative members prepared to "retail" the new knowledge, which in this case included the initial trainer, lead consultant, and senior doctors, nurses, and clinical manager

(3) a supportive practice environment, including in this case librarian, and Trust support for ongoing training, database and computer purchase, and maintenance. Without any one of these elements, each of which requires strategic coordination of people and resources, it is most unlikely that Dr Franks' team would be able systematically to implement research findings appropriately.

To these three elements we would add a fourth, borrowed from anthropological literature,[8] namely "local knowledge" – the local practices, values, and beliefs into which new knowledge must usually be integrated

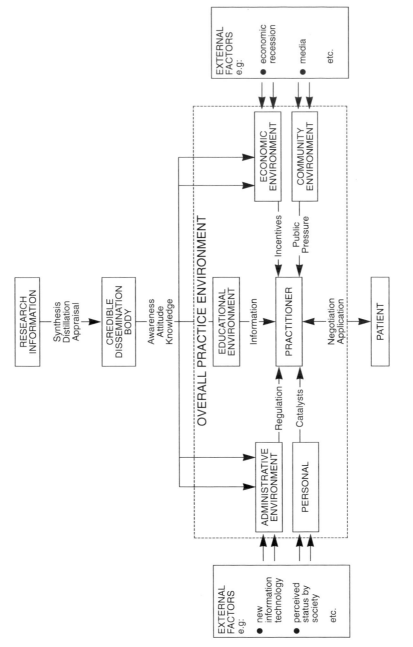

Figure 7.1 The coordinated implementation model

– or risk being rejected. Our experience suggests that systematic use of research findings in clinical practice requires a detailed understanding of the needs and environment of the practitioners in question, and that therefore each firm's strategy must be developed by firm members themselves. For example, the location of the computer, the structure and content of training, and the allocation of ward round, meeting, or audit time to use critical appraisal skills need all to be decided upon by team members who alone know what they need at any particular time.

Undoubtedly, however, some needs are common to most hospital firms. Chapter 10 describes how inadequate attention to common potential barriers, such as inadequate skilling of local users, time-consuming bureaucratic exigencies, inadequate information systems, and policy disincentives to implementing research findings in practice, can all result in the failure of otherwise laudable changes in practice. In our experience, addressing these factors, which usually occur at different levels of the health

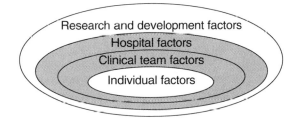

Figure 7.2 Factors affecting the use of research findings in practice usually occur at different levels.

care delivery process (Figure 7.2; Box 7.3), was critical to the success of the firms' projects. Encouragement from management and senior medical staff of the project, time being freed up for clinicians to attend training and implement new problem-solving methods, the use and development of high quality and locally relevant guidelines, readily available sources of information well supported by library and IT staff, and few bureaucratic requirements for organising training and installing databases were common to firms that completed and continued to research findings. Conversely, those firms that delayed or abandoned the project did so for organisational, management-related reasons. These included seniors being too busy to organise and attend training sessions or unenthusiastic about the notion of evidence based practice and therefore providing no role model for juniors; information sources being too difficult to access (for example, no databases being available within a five-minute walk from the worksite); bureaucratic rules about which type of staff would be allowed to access databases (in

Box 7.3   Factors that affect the use of research findings in clinical practice

	Individual and team factors	**Hospital and research and development factors**
Enhancing factors	• Dedicated, confident leadership • Ward-based, high speed computing equipment • Good quality databases relevant to the specialty • Time and staff support for adaptation period (for example, locums to cover regular staff during training) • Some flexibility in the project to allow team ownership and incremental change • Good relationships between medical and nursing staff • Good quality training relevant to team needs for information • Reasonable keyboard and computing skills	• Services to provide research findings when and where needed: databases, librarian and computing support, document delivery system • Information strategy at hospital level or above • Sustained support for lead clinicians (for example, money for training, equipment, and the development of supra-team projects such as guidelines development; encouragement; coordination with other teams and services) • Good quality training: location; relevance to team needs; sustainability • Good salesmanship and on-site assistance from initiator of project (if external to the clinical team)
Barriers	• Uncommitted leader: overworked; uncertain about benefits; threatened by new approach • Insufficient external support for training and managing change (money, time, onsite assistance) • Inadequate computing equipment and databases • Poor relationships between medical and nursing staff • Poor keyboard and computing skills	• Inadequate availability of research findings: patchy, expensive, non-user-friendly databases; slow or non-existent document delivery system; poor computing and librarian support • Lack of management commitment to lead clinician(s) • Lack of time and resources allocated for ongoing training and adaptation of services around the use of research findings • Poor training programmes: irrelevant to team interests; one-off approach; impractical to attend

some hospitals, only academic staff are licensed to use databases; service NHS staff are not included in the software site licence); no mechanisms to allow juniors to obtain bleep-free training sessions; and lack of Trust strategies to support those seniors who were enthusiastic but too overburdened with service work to concentrate on developing decision making capacity in their firms.

Our experience suggests that training should not disrupt existing schedules and hence is best held on-site. On-site training also reinforces the message that quality assurance activities should be an integral part of practice, not a one-off activity performed externally by "experts". Training was most effective when it addressed staff's current needs for information and trainers could discuss suitable teaching materials from the outset in collaboration with team leaders. In addition, interactive teaching methods have widely been found to be most effective, enabling learners to refine skills and knowledge that they already possess rather than lecture-based teaching that presents evidence based practice as an elaborate and alien concept, discouraging newcomers to medical research and epidemiology. Computer equipment must be both secure and readily accessible for busy staff and databases must run quickly, requiring a computer with adequate specifications and maintenance. Existing activities should be harnessed for practising searching and appraising skills, such as journal club meetings, firm and hospital meetings, and ward-rounds, rather than forcing already stretched practitioners to make extra time. Finally, Trust support is ultimately needed for the maintenance of evidence based practice through the development of library services, the ongoing allocation of time for training, and investment in computing equipment. Such support is an important morale boost to busy clinicians attempting to make major changes to their decision making environments. In this case study, Dr Franks could probably have done more to include Trust board members in the project, for instance by inviting them to an "evidence based ward round" and discussing the potential of evidence based practice to the Trust.

However, despite the predictability of many firm needs, Dr Franks' example would suggest that imbuing key decisions with the firm's own local knowledge is critical to gain the credibility, consent, and commitment required to make such changes successful. As Lomas points out, the joint decision making entailed requires considerable coordination,[7] but in our experience, the pay-off is worth it. When allowed to do so, firms have successfully undertaken evidence based practice in a number of diverse and unforeseen ways, from individual patient care decisions to the development of guidelines and the improvement of local purchasing decisions, accurately reflecting and addressing their different needs and resources.

Acknowledgements

The authors would like to acknowledge all the consultants and their staff whom we have trained over the past three years, including the 18 firms who participated in the North Thames "Front-line Evidence based Medicine Project", for making the case study in this article possible. This case study is not based on any single individual or team.

References

1 Milne R, Donald A, Chambers L. Piloting short workshops on the critical appraisal of reviews. *Health Trends*. 1995;27:120–3.
2 Booth A. *The ScHARR guide to evidence based practice*. Sheffield: School of Health and Related Research Information Services, 1996.
3 Critical Appraisal Skills Programme. *Orientation guide 1996*. Oxford: Institute of Health Sciences, 1996.
4 Counsell C, Sandercock P. The efficacy and safety of anticoagulant therapy in patients with acute presumed ischaemic stroke: a systematic review of the randomised trials comparing anticoagulants with controls. In: Warlow C, van Gijn J, Sandercock P. ed. *Stroke Module of The Cochrane Database of Systematic Reviews* [upated 3 June 1996]. Available in The Cochrane Library [database on disk and CD-ROM]; The Cochrane Collaboration, Issue 2; Oxford: Update Software, 1996. Updated quarterly. Available from: BMJ Publishing Group, London.
5 Gray JAM. *Evidence based healthcare*. London: Churchill Livingstone, 1996.
6 Straus S, Sackett DL. Using research findings in clinical practice. *BMJ*.
7 Lomas J. Retailing research: increasing the role of evidence in clinical services for childbirth. *Milbank Q* 1993;71(3):439–76.
8 Geertz C. *Local Knowledge: further essays in interpretive anthropology*. New York: Basic Books, 1983.

8 Using research findings in clinical practice

S E STRAUS AND D L SACKETT

Introduction

In clinical practice, caring for patients generates many questions about diagnosis, prognosis, and therapy which challenges us to keep up to date with the medical literature. In a study of North American general physicians, it was found that two clinically important questions arose for every three patients seen.[1] Another challenge to keeping abreast of the medical literature is the volume of clinical literature. As general physicians who want to keep up to date with journals relevant to our practice, we face the task of examining 19 articles a day, 365 days a year.[2]

One approach to meeting these challenges and avoiding clinical entropy is to learn how to practise evidence based medicine. The practice of evidence based medicine involves integrating individual clinical expertise with the best available clinical evidence from systematic research.[3] Individual clinical expertise implies the proficiency and judgement that individual clinicians acquire through clinical experience and clinical practice. Best available clinical evidence is defined as clinically relevant research, which may be from the basic sciences of medicine but especially from patient-centred clinical research into the accuracy and precision of diagnostic tests, precision of prognostic markers, and the efficacy and safety of therapeutic, rehabilitative, and preventive regimens.[3] This chapter will focus on what evidence based medicine is and how it can be practised by the busy clinician.

The practice of evidence based medicine is a process of lifelong, self-directed learning in which caring for our patients creates the need for clinically important information about diagnosis, prognosis, therapy, and

63

other health care issues. Box 8.1 illustrates the five steps involved in practising evidence based medicine which allow us to fulfil these needs.

Box 8.1   The five steps of evidence based medicine

1 Convert information needs into clinically relevant, answerable questions.
2 Track down, with maximum efficiency, the best evidence with which to answer these questions (whether from the clinical examination, the diagnostic laboratory, published research, or other sources).
3 Critically appraise the evidence for its validity (closeness to the truth) and usefulness (clinical applicability).
4 Integrate this appraisal with our clinical expertise and apply the results in our clinical practice.
5 Evaluate our performance.

Asking answerable clinical questions

Formulating clear, focused clinical questions is a prerequisite for answering them, and this requires specifying their four elements:

(1) the patient or problem being addressed
(2) the intervention, whether by nature or by clinical design (a cause, prognostic factor, treatment, etc.), being considered
(3) a comparison intervention, when relevant
(4) the clinical outcome or outcomes of interest.[4]

To illustrate how many questions can arise from a patient scenario, consider a 65-year-old man with a history of cirrhosis secondary to alcohol abuse who presents to Accident and Emergency with confusion and increasing abdominal girth. He is on a diuretic and had been hospitalised two months earlier with spontaneous bacterial peritonitis. On examination, he is disoriented and jaundiced but afebrile, with a blood pressure of 110/60 and a heart rate of 80 beats per minute. In addition to spider nevi and gynaecomastia, he has tense ascites and a tender abdomen, but bowel sounds are present.

Dozens of questions can arise as we try to help this patient, and some of them are summarised in Box 8.2. Note that they include a wide array of issues for clinical findings, aetiology, differential diagnosis, diagnostic tests, prognosis, therapy, prevention, and self-improvement.[4] Given their breadth and number, and admitting that we are likely to have only about 30 minutes in the next week to address any of them,[5] we pare all of these down to just one question by balancing the question that would be most

Box 8.2   Examples of clinical questions that arise from our patient

- Clinical findings: In a patient with suspected ascites, which is the most accurate and precise way of diagnosing ascites on physical examination – fluid wave or shifting dullness?
- Aetiology: In a patient with ascites secondary to cirrhosis and suspected spontaneous bacterial peritonitis, can spontaneous bacterial peritonitis cause confusion?
- Differential diagnosis: In a patient with ascites secondary to cirrhosis, which is the most likely to cause increased ascites – spontaneous bacterial peritonitis or a change in diuretic?
- Diagnostic tests: In a patient with suspected alcohol abuse, is the use of the CAGE* questionnaire specific for diagnosing alcohol abuse?
- Prognosis: In a patient with cirrhosis, ascites, and spontaneous bacterial peritonitis, does spontaneous bacterial peritonitis increase his mortality?
- Therapy: When performing a paracentesis on a patient with ascites secondary to cirrhosis, does intravenous albumin prevent circulatory dysfunction?
- Prevention: Does prophylaxis with antibiotics in a patient with cirrhosis and ascites decrease the risk of spontaneous bacterial peritonitis and mortality?
- Self-improvement: In order to improve my understanding of the pathophysiology of ascites, would I gain more from spending an hour going to the library and reading a textbook or spending 15 minutes on the ward computer looking at the CD version of the same textbook?

Am J Med 1987;**82**:231.

important to our patient's well being against that which appears most feasible to answer, is most interesting to us, and is most likely to be raised again in subsequent patients. For our patient, we decide to focus on the question: in a patient with cirrhosis and ascites, does prophylactic treatment with antibiotics decrease the risk of spontaneous bacterial peritonitis and mortality?

Searching for the best evidence

A focused question sharpens our search for the best evidence. Searching tips for increasing sensitivity and specificity of this search have been developed by teams of research librarians and clinicians, and can be found in a variety of paper[4] and electronic[6] sites; local librarians also can be extremely helpful in guiding and assisting our searches.

65

The types and numbers of evidence resources are rapidly expanding and some of them have already undergone critical appraisal in their creation. Most rigorous of these are the systematic reviews of the effects of health care generated by the Cochrane Collaboration, readily available as the Cochrane Library[8] on compact disk and accompanied by abstracts for critically appraised overviews in the Database of Abstracts of Reviews of Effectiveness created by the York Centre for Reviews and Dissemination. The former are exhaustive and therefore take years to generate; the latter can be generated in months. Still faster is the appearance of clinical articles about diagnosis, prognosis, therapy, quality of care, and economics that pass both specific methodological standards (such that their results are likely to be valid) and clinical scrutiny for relevance (this two-stage selection reduces the clinical literature by 98%), and appear in "evidence based" journals such as *ACP Journal Club*, *Evidence based Medicine* and *Evidence based Cardiovascular Medicine*. In these journals, the evidence is summarised in structured abstracts, and one of several hundred clinical experts adds a commentary to each which provides the clinical expertise necessary to place it in context.

These journals can be searched and read in a problem-solving mode. An electronic publication, Best Evidence, combines all six years of *ACP Journal Club* and the contents of *Evidence based Medicine* in an easily searched compact disk.[8] Searching Best Evidence for spontaneous bacterial peritonitis and cirrhosis brought up the abstract and commentary for a trial of prophylaxis against recurrent spontaneous bacterial peritonitis with trimethoprim-sulphamethoxazole.[9]

In addition, some evidence based materials are now appearing on the Internet, including those of the Cochrane Collaboration,[10] and some sites include clinically useful evidence about diagnosis, prognosis, and therapy. (Our site in Oxford permits browsers to apply the specificity of shifting dullness and the sensitivity of a history of ankle swelling in sorting out patients thought to have ascites, which can be used to answer some of the questions in Box 8.2.[6]) If the foregoing rapid, evidence based medicine access strategies fail, we resort to the time-honoured and increasingly friendly systems for accessing the current literature via MEDLINE and EMBASE, employing methodological quality filters to maximise the yield of high quality evidence.[6]

Critically appraising the evidence

Once we find potentially useful evidence, we have to critically appraise it and determine if it is valid and useful. Guides have been generated to help us evaluate the validity of evidence about a diagnostic test (was there an independent, blind comparison with a gold standard of diagnosis?), a treatment (was the assignment of patients to treatments really randomised?), a prognostic marker (was an appropriate sample of patients assembled at a uniform point in their illness?), or a guideline or other strategy for improving the quality of care we give our patients,[4,11] and worksheets for applying them are also available.[6] With the advent of the "more informative abstract", we find that many of the guides can be answered from reading it. Assessing the article we found on prophylaxis against spontaneous bacterial peritonitis, we decide it is valid and the results show that trimethoprim-sulphamethoxazole decreases the risk of peritonitis significantly. While there was a trend for decrease in mortality in the group treated with antibiotics, this was not statistically significant which may be a function of insufficient power.

After we have gone to the trouble of finding an article and determining if its results are valid and useful, it often would be helpful to file our summary so that we can refer to it again or pass it along to colleagues or other learners. One way to do this is to prepare a one-page summary of the patient, the evidence, and the clinical "bottom line", organised as a "critically appraised topic" or CAT.[12] CAT makers (for constructing, calculating, storing, and printing CATs) are becoming available, as are websites for their storage and retrieval;[6] we suggest that they are more useful to their producers (we become more effective and efficient in searching and critically appraising) than to potential users (since CATs undergo little peer review and may be useful mainly for their citations).

Applying the evidence

Applying the results of our critical appraisals involves the essential second element of evidence based medicine: integrating the evidence with our own clinical expertise and our knowledge of the unique features of our patients and their predicaments, rights, and expectations; only then can we decide whether and how to incorporate the evidence into their care. Returning to our patient, we found from the paper that the evidence favouring treatment with trimethoprim-sulphamethoxazole was valid although we are less certain about its effects on mortality and the side-effects associated with its use. Accordingly, the decision whether to use it would have to grow out of a "therapeutic alliance" with our patient who was informed about the potential risks as well as benefits of this therapy. This involves discussing with the patient his preferences, concerns, and expectations about both risks and benefits of treatment.

Evaluation of our performance

Evaluation of our performance of these four steps to evidence based medicine completes the cycle. We can evaluate our progress through each stage of asking answerable questions (were they?), searching for the best evidence (did we find good evidence quickly?), critical appraisal (did we do so effectively and efficiently?), and integrating the appraisal with our clinical expertise and our patient's unique features (did we end up with a rational, acceptable management strategy?). This fifth step of self-evaluation allows you to focus on earlier steps that need improvement in the future. We can assess our application of the evidence we found about prophylactic treatment of spontaneous bacterial peritonitis – did we discuss the risks and benefits of treatment and incorporate the patient's own values into our discussion?

Conclusions

Can medical practice be evidence based? Recent audits have been encouraging, as when a general medicine service at a university-affiliated district general hospital documented that 53% of the undiagnosed patients admitted to it received primary treatments that had been validated in randomised trials or systematic review of randomised trials (an additional 29% of patients received care based on convincing non-experimental evidence).[13] Three-quarters of this evidence was immediately available in the form of previously generated CATs, and the remaining quarter was identified and applied through immediately (at the time of admission) asking answerable questions, rapidly finding good evidence, quickly determining its validity and usefulness, swiftly integrating it with clinical expertise and unique patient features, and offering it to the patients at once. Similar results have been found in a study performed at a psychiatric hospital,[14] general practitioners' office,[15] and a paediatric surgery department.[16]

In sum, practising evidence based medicine is one way for us to keep up to date with the exponentially growing medical literature, not just by more efficient "browsing" but by improving our skills in asking answerable questions, finding the best evidence, critically appraising it, integrating it with our clinical expertise and our patients' unique features, and applying the results in our clinical practice. When added to conscientiously practised clinical skills and constantly developing clinical expertise, sound external evidence can efficiently and effectively be brought to bear on our patients' problems.

References

1 Covell DG, Uman GC, Manning PR. Information needs in office practice: are they being met? *Ann Intern Med* 1985;**103**:596–9.

2 Davidoff F, Haynes RB, Sackett DL, Smith R. Evidence based medicine: a new journal to help doctors identify the information they need. *BMJ* 1995;**310**:1085–6.

3 Sackett DL, Rosenberg WMC, Gray JAM, Richardson WS. Evidence based medicine: what it is and what it isn't. *BMJ* 1996;**312**:71–2.

4 Sackett DL, Richardson WS, Rosenberg WMC, Haynes RB. *Evidence based medicine: how to practice and teach EBM*. London: Churchill Livingstone, 1997.

5 Sackett DL. Using evidence based medicine to help physicians keep up to date. *Serials* 1996;**9**:178–81.

6 NHS R&D Centre for Evidence based Medicine in Oxford, UK. Uniform Resource Locator: hffp://cebm.jr2.ox.act.uk/.

7 Cochrane Collaboration. Cochrane Database of Systematic Reviews, 2nd issue. London: BMJ Publishing Group, 1995.

8 Best Evidence. London: BMJ Publishing Group, 1996.

9 Reichen J. Commentary on trimethoprim-sulfamethoxazole for the prevention of spontaneous bacterial peritonitis in cirrhosis. *ACP J Club* 1995;**123**:42.

10 Cochrane Collaboration. Uniform Resource Locator: http://hiru.mcmaster.ca/COCHRANE.

11 Oxman AD, Sackett DL, Guyatt GH for the Evidence based Medicine Working Group User's guides to the medical literature. I. How to get started. The Evidence Based Medicine Working Group. *JAMA* 1993;**270**:2093–5.

12 Sauve JS, Lee HM, Farkouh ME, Sackett DL. The critically appraised topic: a practical approach to learning critical appraisal. *Ann Roy Coll Phys Surg Canada* 1995;**28**:396–8.

13 Ellis J. Mulligan I, Rower J. Sackett DL. In-patient general medicine is evidence based. *Lancet* 1995;**346**:407–10.

14 Geddes JR, Game D, Jenkins NE, Peterson LA, Pottinger GR, Sackett DL. What proportion of primary psychiatric interventions are based on randomised evidence? *Qual Health Care* 1996;**5**:215–17.

15 Gill P, Dowell AC, Neal RP, Smith N, Heywood P, Wilson AK. Evidence based general practice: a retrospective study of interventions in our training practice. *BMJ* 1996;**312**: 819 21.

16 Kenny SE, Shankar KR, Rentala R, Lamont GL, Lloyd DA. Evidence based surgery: interventions in a regional paediatric surgical unit. *Arch Dis Child* 1997;**76**(1):50–3.

9 Evidence based policy making

J A MUIR GRAY

A policy is defined in the *Shorter Oxford English Dictionary* as "a course of action adopted and pursued by a government, party, ruler, statesman; any course of action adopted as advantageous or expedient".

The term "policy" by itself is inevitably closely associated with politics and politicians although the term is now used in other ways, for example as "managerial policy" or "clinical policy". In this broader definition a policy may be defined as "a course of action that an authority states should be followed".

Politics, from the same root, is defined in the *Shorter Oxford English Dictionary* as "relating to the principles, opinions, or sympathies of a person or party". Thus political decisions are based upon values and beliefs as well as being based on evidence, and it is possible to represent the three main factors that influence policy making in a Venn diagram (Figure 9.1).

Different types of values influence policy makers. Some of these values are general values related to prevailing ideological beliefs. These values may sometimes be presented as polar opposites but they are often on a continuum. For example, one analysis of policy making in Canada and the United States considered the impact that different political philosophies in the two countries placed on the relative importance of evidence, with the United States focusing on the rights of individuals to make decisions whereas Canadian policy making was influenced by the values of solidarity and community benefit.[1] A clear example of the application of this philosophy is illustrated by the decisions that have been taken in the United States on mammographic screening for women under 50.

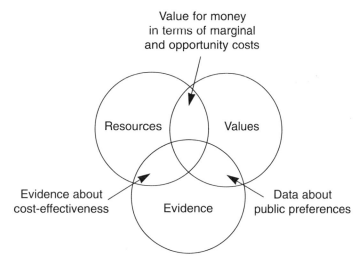

Figure 9.1 Venn diagram showing the three main factors that influence policy making: resources, values, and evidence.

The *Alice in Wonderland* of breast cancer screening

The name "Bethesda" is revered in the scientific community not for its religious connotations but because it is the place where the National Institutes of Health (NIH) are based in a huge sprawling campus with its own underground station and bus service.

The NIH Consensus Conference concluded that routine mammography was not indicated for women in their forties, but when the Consensus Conference reached this evidence based decision[2] the press savagely attacked the decision and the panel of experts convened by the NIH accusing them of condemning women to death. The *New York Times* and Congress made up their own minds and called for screening to be introduced.

Values dominate in Bethesda

The Director of the National Cancer Institute, one of the Institutes of the NIH, said that he was "shocked" by the report[3] and asked the Institute's 18-member Advisory Board to review the evidence; they voted by 17 to 1 to recommend the introduction of screening for women under 50.[4]

In neither Canada nor the United Kingdom has a decision been made to introduce mammographic screening for women under 50 as a routine. Those who defend this policy would argue that it was solely evidence based but a perspective from the United States might be that the use of evidence

71

in a country in which a decision had been made to allocate a finite amount of resources to health care was always influenced by the impact that limited resources had on decision making.

In the United States, advice about mammographic screening can be promulgated with the decision being left to the individual woman who will include this in their insurance coverage or pay for the mammographic screening themselves, basing the decision on advice emanating from their country's most respected clinical research centre. The fact that this advice will be irrelevant for many poor people is not a factor in the United States' decision because health care is an individual responsibility, whereas in the United Kingdom, where health is considered to be both a community and an individual responsibility, any benefit enjoyed by a small number of people who may be helped by screening would have to be offset by the impact that such a decision would have on the finite amount of resources available and other people who would have to "pay" for the introduction of mammographic screening in women under 50.

Health and health service policies

A wide variety of different policies to improve the health of populations are made by governments but they may be divided into two main types – health policies and health care policies. Health policies are designed to promote and protect health and have a direct bearing on the health of the populations governed. Some would argue that any policy will have an impact on health, for example a policy that successfully creates wealth will improve health, as has happened in Japan and the other successful economies of the Pacific rim; but by convention industrial policies are not usually classified as health policies, which are restricted to those measures primarily designed to promote and protect health.

In the United Kingdom a Minister of public health has been appointed to ensure that the health implications of all government policies are considered.

Different standards of evidence for health promotion and health protection

Protecting individuals from harm by third parties is a traditional role of the State and policies to protect the health of individuals or groups, for example environmental policies to prevent pollution, are usually less strongly opposed and may require a lower level of strength of evidence than health promotion policies. In three masterly essays, Lord Ashby, formerly the Chair of the Royal Commission on Environmental Pollution, described the way in which factors other than the strength of evidence affected the decision making threshold.[5] In this book he tells how a few dramatic pieces in the newspaper were of apparently much greater impact than the deliberations of the Royal Commission.

Health promotion policies are designed to protect the health of individuals. This type of legislation, though now commonplace in many countries, is often resisted because of a deep-seated opposition to paternalistic legislation, and therefore requires much stronger evidence before it can be introduced. Furthermore, paternalistic legislation designed to protect a minority may result in harm to one of those who are not protected by the measure introduced by legislation. This was a crucial issue in the debate before seat-belts were made compulsory in the United Kingdom. Opponents of seat-belt legislation argued not only that it was ethically wrong for the State to force individuals to do anything for their own good, using the trenchant prose of J S Mill's essay *On Liberty*[6] to support their argument; they also produced evidence that individuals were harmed as a result of wearing seat-belts, for example by being unable to get clear of a car in water or on fire. The evidence for the protective effect of seat-belts was strong, but the evidence suggesting that some people would be harmed so that others might live was emotive, and it was not until yet more evidence was produced that the main reason why individuals were unable to escape from crashes was not the wearing of a seat-belt but the unconsciousness that resulted from failing to wear a seat belt that the argument started to turn.

It is important in this context to emphasise that different standards are used in passing legislation and promoting policies to protect children. The United States has introduced a number of measures to control smoking, ostensibly to benefit children, but these same measures will also be helpful to adults.

Health care policies

Health care policies govern the funding and organisation of health services. Policy is very often linked to finance, for the direction of finance to a given end is one means by which policymakers can ensure that their policies are put into practice. Apart from the decision about how much money should go to health care, as opposed to transport or education or defence, almost all decisions which affect finance result in a reorganisation of a service, for policy making is not simply concerned with switching money between, for example, cancer services and cardiac services but with ways in which the money is controlled and decisions are made. Thus the introduction of GP fundholding in the United Kingdom was not simply a means of shifting money from one part of the service to another; it had profound constitutional effects on the way in which the service was organised and managed.

Health care policies can affect the organisation of a service without affecting the flow of finance. For example, the introduction of Community Health Councils in 1974 was a change in organisation which influenced rather than caused a change in the management of the resources but reflected the political value ascribed to consumer involvement.

The introduction of new health *care* policies is less often evidence based than the introduction of new health policies. One reason for this is that health service research is often less generalisable than health research. For example, experiments with health maintenance organisations in the United States are less easy to generalise from than research on new vaccines.

Evidence-driven policy decisions

There are very clear examples where the production of new evidence has led to a new policy. A paper in the *Lancet* describing the effectiveness of a breast screening programme in Sweden was of interest to the House of Commons and led to the development of a national committee, the Forrest Committee (REF), which reviewed the evidence on breast cancer screening, and to the recommendation that breast cancer screening be introduced as a national screening service.[7] This whole process took place over the course of less than three years.

Resource-driven policy decisions

The Venn diagram shown in Figure 9.1 emphasises the importance of resources in policy making, for policies have to be realisable and deliverable. Pressures on resources, either financial pressures or the shortage of skilled manpower, may create problems and lead to policies being reviewed, although this level of decision making is perhaps more appropriately considered as managerial policy making rather than health care policy making. The former is focused on how the resources allocated to a service or population should be used to best effect; the latter focuses on how decisions are made about resource allocation.

When resources get tight and new options have to be considered, then evidence is assembled to appraise the costs and benefits of the different policy options. This level of policy option appraisal using evidence was developed primarily by economists and terms such as cost–benefit analysis, cost-effectiveness analysis, and decision analysis are increasingly used in policy making both by politicians and by managers.

Cost–benefit analysis is a technique in which evidence about the costs and benefits of various options is gathered and translated into financial terms. This means that what may be very firm evidence, for example about the number of deaths that may result from one option or another, has to be combined with highly judgemental decisions about the value that should be ascribed to a death of an individual depending upon their age and state of health. Cost–benefit analysis thus allows people to compare the benefits of, for example, an immunisation programme or a treatment programme. In cost-effectiveness analysis, the relative costs of achieving the same effects are calculated, for example the cost-effectiveness of renal dialysis and transplantation as a means of preventing death from end-stage renal failure. Fewer judgements have to be made in this type of analysis than in cost–benefit analysis, and it is possible for this type of decision to be based on much firmer evidence. New options for using economic evaluations to promote the uptake of research findings are discussed in chapter 14.

A technique called "decision analysis" is now becoming more popular (see Chapter 12). In decision analysis, for example of different options for screening for Down's syndrome, an algorithm has been developed which shows the effects of different decisions. Usually the algorithm also includes the adoption of value judgements about the beneficial or adverse effects of different options.[8] In all these techniques it is now customary to use sensitivity analysis, for example to determine what would happen to the analysis and its conclusions if any of the variables changed significantly.

Future trends in evidence based policy making

Predicting policy making is hazardous and perhaps unwise. However, two trends can be discerned in all developed countries – increasing pressure on resources and a better educated population, more sceptical about the evidence produced by scientists.[9]

As the pressure on resources increases, driven in the health service by rising expectations, population ageing, and new technology, decision makers will have to face tougher decisions. A better educated population will not only have higher expectations of health and other public services but of the decision making process itself, expecting the decisions to be explicit, open, and evidence based.

The last 50 years has seen a dramatic change in decision making in the UK from an era in which decisions were made by politicians who were primarily lawyers, supported by civil servants who were primarily generalists, particularly in the UK where there was a strong tradition of a Civil Service based on the study of the classics with the scientists within the Civil Service being traditionally accorded lower status. The Second World War changed this, allowing the technocrats to demonstrate what science could do by

75

bringing evidence to decision making; this is brilliantly described in David Halberstam's book *The best and the brightest*.[10] In ministries of health, public health doctors and epidemiologists had brought science and policy making closer together since the latter part of the 19th century but it is only in the last 50 years that evidence based decision making has become common across all areas of policy making.

In the UK a conscious decision was taken by policy-makers to ensure that 1.5 percent of the resources made available for patient care should be invested to support research and development. The main reason for doing this was to improve the quality and effectiveness of health care by producing answers to the questions that health care decision-makers – clinicians, managers and patients – were asking, and by taking explicit steps to ensure that decisions were based on evidence both through using the performance management system to promote clinical effectiveness and by promoting an evaluative culture designed to make decision-makers hungry for best current knowledge which the R&D Programme would provide. This explicit commitment to create an evidence based health care system emphasised the recognition that policy-makers gave to the need for evidence based decision making.

Epidemiologists can be proud of the fact that they were among the first to practise evidence based decision making, analysing patterns of health and disease to identify the causes of ill health, although the interventions they proposed to tackle these causes were often based on inference and not on hard evidence. For the future it seems certain that the tradition of evidence based policy making will become increasingly explicit.

Evidence and value-based decision making

One of the main consequences of promoting evidence based decision making has been the clarification of a distinction between values and evidence. Before evidence based decision making became a powerful paradigm, decisions were made on a combination of opinions and resources. The obsession with identifying evidence has led to an explosion of the concept of the opinion, with the two different elements of the opinion, propositions supported by evidence and value judgement, now being much more clearly exposed. Thus the move to evidence based decision making has also led to values becoming much more explicit and exposed.

In future decisions will not simply be decisions about whether or not to fund a new intervention or stop an existing intervention. Health care decision making does not take place on a blank sheet of paper. All health care budgets are fully committed and decisions always take place at the margins. Thus the values that will be exposed are those which are exposed when change is made at the margin. The decision whether or not to increase investment in, for example, Down's Syndrome screening will inevitably raise issues about where the money is to be found to make that increased investment. Should it come from within the budget for antenatal services, and, if so, what are the values that should be used to decide on areas for disinvestment?

Alternatively, should it come from some other health care programme, for example by reducing the amount of money spent on hip replacement, coronary artery bypass grafting, or some other intervention for older people? This would again expose the values that have to be addressed in shifting resources from one group in the population to another.

The analysis of evidence has opened one black box in health care decisions; in doing so it has revealed another black box, the black box of values and preferences, and it is this aspect of decision making that will dominate the next phase of evidence based policy-making.

Acknowledgements

I am grateful to Emily Gray for her help with the concepts of J S Mill.

References

1 Tanenbaum SJ. *"Medical effectiveness" in Canadian and US health policy: the comparative politics of inferential ambiguity. Health Serv Res* 1996;**31**:5, 517–32.
2 National Cancer Institute. *National Institutes of Health consensus statement: Breast cancer screening for women aged 40–49.* Bethesda, MD: NIH, 1997.
3 Marwick C. *NIH consensus panel spurs discontent. JAMA* 1997;**277**:519–20.
4 Fletcher SW. *Whither scientific deliberation in health policy recommendations? Alice in the Wonderland of breast-cancer screening. New Eng J Med* 1997;**336**:1180–3.
5 Ashby, the Lord. *Reconciling man and the environment.* Oxford University Press, 1978.
6 Mill JS. *On Liberty.* Fontana Library, 1969.
7 Forrest P. *Breast cancer screening.* Report of a working group of the Department of Health, 1986.
8 Fletcher J, Hicks NR, Kay JDS, Body PA. *Using decision analysis to compare policies for antenatal screening for Down's syndrome. BMJ* 1996;**311**:351–6.
9 Angell, M. *Science on Trial.* New York: WW Norton & Co. Inc., 1996.
10 Halberstam D. *The best and the brightest.* Random House, 1986.

10 Barriers and bridges to evidence based clinical practice

BRIAN HAYNES AND ANDREW HAINES

Introduction

Clinicians and health care planners seeking to improve the quality and efficiency of health services can find help from evidence from health care research. This evidence is increasingly accessible through information services combining high quality evidence with information technology. But there are several important barriers to the successful application of evidence from research. This chapter will outline both the prospects for harnessing evidence to improve health care and the problems that readers – clinicians, planners, and patients – will need to overcome to enjoy the benefits (Box 10.1).

The aim of evidence based health care is to provide the means by which current best evidence from research can be judiciously and conscientiously applied in the prevention, detection, and care of human health disorders.[1] This aim is decidedly ambitious, given how slowly important new treatments disseminate into practice[2-4] and how resistant existing treatments that have been disproved are to being removed from practice.[5]

The barriers to dissemination and timely application of evidence in health care decision making are complex and little studied. They include many factors beyond the control of the practitioner and patient (such as being in the wrong place when illness comes) as well as factors that might be modified to advantage (such as doing the wrong thing at the right time). Rather than attempt to dissect all these barriers, we present a simple path (Figure 10.1) along which evidence might travel to assist with health care decisions in a timely way. We will consider both some barriers along this path and some bridges that are being constructed over the barriers.

78

Box 10.1 Some barriers to evidence based clinical practice and some solutions

Barriers

- The size and noise of the research enterprise
- Problems in developing evidence based clinical policy
- Difficulties in applying evidence in practice, including
  - poor access to current best evidence and guidelines
  - organisational barriers
  - ineffectual continuing education
  - low patient adherence to treatments

Solutions

- Research abstraction and synthesis services
- Guidelines for guidelines
- Information systems that integrate evidence and guidelines with patient care
- Facilities and incentives for effective care; disease management systems
- Effective continuing education and quality improvement programmes for practitioners
- Effective strategies to assist patients to follow evidence based health care advice

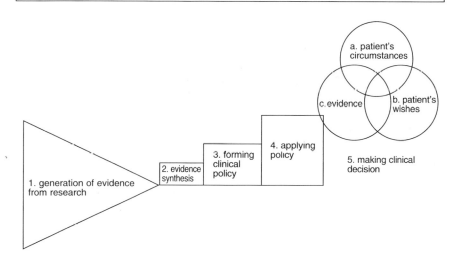

Figure 10.1 Path from evidence generation to clinical application

The research wedge (step 1)

The path begins (see Figure 10.1, step 1) with a wedge that represents biomedical research, the process of testing innovations in health care, eliminating those that lack merit (thus, the shape of the wedge). Testing of innovations begins at the broad edge of the wedge, usually in laboratories, with many new products and processes being discarded on early testing. Those with merit in early testing then undergo field trials in humans, these studies being first aimed at assessing major toxicity, then at estimating efficacy. Again, many innovations fail, but a few merit more definitive testing in large controlled trials with major clinical end-points. It is only when studies show success at the tip of the wedge that major efforts at dissemination and application are warranted. Increasingly, behavioural interventions, surgical procedures, and alternative approaches to the organization and delivery of care are being subjected to similarly rigorous evaluation.

The biomedical and applied research enterprise represented by the wedge is vigorous, with an annual investment of over US$ 55 billion annually around the world,[6] giving rise to the hope that health care can be improved despite cutbacks in health service spending in many countries. Unfortunately, many loose connections exist between the research effort and clinical practice, not the least of which is that preliminary studies far outnumber definitive ones, and all compete in the medical literature for the attention of readers.[7]

Steps from research to practice

The boxes following the wedge in Figure 10.1 (steps 2–4) represent three steps that are needed to harness research evidence for health care practice. These steps include 2 – getting the evidence straight, 3 – developing clinical policy from the evidence, and 4 – applying the policy at the right place, way, and time. All three steps must be negotiated to form a valid connection between evidence and practice.

Getting the evidence straight (step 2)

Most news from research appears first in peer-reviewed journals, but the small number of clinically important studies are thinly spread throughout a huge literature, so that individual readers are bound to be overwhelmed. Skills in critical appraisal of evidence have been developed and disseminated for some time[8] but applying these is time-consuming. The newest bridges for this barrier include abstract services that apply principles of critical appraisal to select studies that are ready for clinical application, and independently summarize these studies.[9,10] Many more of these "new breed" journals are in development so that eventually most major clinical specialties will have their own. More important, the Cochrane Collaboration has pledged to summarise all sound trials of health care interventions and the Cochrane Library is now a robust resource.[11]

Along with these new services, advances in information technology now provide quick and often very inexpensive access to high quality health care evidence from the bedside, office, and home.[8,12] Computerised decision support systems are now maturing and taking evidence one step further, working it into patient-specific reminders and decision aids embedded in clinical information systems (see Chapter 11).[13] These innovations are making evidence based health care much more feasible.

Creating evidence based clinical policy (step 3)

To be both evidence based and clinically useful, clinical policy must carefully balance the strengths and limitations of all relevant research evidence with the practical realities of the health care and clinical setting.[14] This is a problematic step at present because of limitations in both evidence and policy making. Clinical practice guidelines derived by national groups can help individual practitioners, but the expertise, will, resources, and effort required to make them scientifically sound as well as clinically helpful are in short supply, as witnessed by conflicting guidelines from various august bodies.[15] National health care policies are often moulded by a range of non-research factors, including historical, cultural, and ideological influences. Moreover, when national guidelines or health care policies exhort clinicians to perform acts that are not evidence based, this unnecessary work acts as a barrier to implementation of well-founded knowledge. "Guidelines for guidelines" have been developed that will help if followed.[16]

Evidence and guidelines must be understood by practitioners if they are to be well applied, a slow process that is not much aided by traditional continuing education offerings.[17] Further, local and individual clinical practice circumstances often vary for the delivery of care, and national guidelines must be tailored for local circumstances by local practitioners if they are to be applied, a process that is only just beginning to occur.[18] Evidence can be used directly by individual practitioners to make policies, but few practitioners have the time and skill to do so. The difficulties in developing sound policies are perhaps the greatest barriers to implementation of research findings at present. Clinicians are in the best position to be able to balance research evidence with clinical circumstances, and must think and act as part of the planning team if progress is to be made.

Applying evidence based policy in practice (step 4)

The next step from research to practice is to apply evidence based policy at the right time and place and in the right way. Again there are barriers at the local and individual clinical levels. For example, for thrombolysis for acute myocardial infarction to be delivered within its brief time window of efficacy, the patient must recognise the symptoms, get to the hospital (avoiding a potentially delaying call to her family physician), and be seen right away by a health professional who recognises the problem and initiates treatment. For many people in many places, this is still not happening.[19,20]

In some cases, particularly for surgery and other skilled procedures, lack of training constitutes a barrier. The complexity of guidelines may also thwart their application.[21] Organisational barriers to change must also be dealt with, for example ensuring that general practitioners have access to echocardiography for the diagnosis of heart failure before starting angiotensin-converting enzyme inhibitors.[22] Changes in the organisation of care, including disease management, improvements in continuing education and quality improvement interventions for practitioners,[17] and advances in computerised decision support systems,[13] are beginning to make inroads into these last steps of connecting research evidence with practice. Unfortunately, these may all be undermined by limitations in resources for health services, and the use of inappropriate economic measures for evaluating health care programmes[23] when cost-effective interventions may require considerable upfront investment with delayed benefits, as is especially true for preventive procedures.

Making clinical decisions (step 5)

Once the evidence has been delivered to the practitioner and the practitioner has recalled the evidence correctly and at the right place and time, there are still steps to be taken. First, the practitioner must determine the patient's unique circumstances: what is wrong and how is it affecting this patient? For example, the cost-effectiveness of lowering cholesterol with statins is highly dependent on the patient's own risk of adverse outcomes.[24] What other problems is the patient suffering from that might bear on which treatments are likely to be safe and effective? For example, carotid endarterectomy is highly effective for symptomatic, tight carotid stenosis[25] but patients must be surgically fit to receive it. Sizing up the patient's clinical circumstances is the domain of clinical expertise, without which no amount of evidence from research will suffice.

Also, and increasingly, the patient's preferences, values, and rights are entering into the process of deciding on the appropriate management. Thus, patients who are averse to immediate risk or cost may decline surgical procedures that offer longer-term benefits, including endarterectomy, even if they are surgically fit. Evidence from research must be integrated with the patient's clinical circumstances and wishes to derive a meaningful decision about management, a process that no "cookbook" can describe. Indeed, we are still ignorant about the art of clinical practice. Although there is some evidence that exploring patients' experiences of illness may lead to improvements in their outcomes,[26] the topic of improving communication between clinician and patient is in need of major research efforts if we are to enhance progress in achieving evidence based health care. Meanwhile, there is a growing body of information for patients that is both scientifically sound and intelligible, and many consumer and patient groups have made such material widely available.[27] Interactive media are being employed (but are not widely deployed) to assist patients with diagnostic and treatment choices.[28]

Finally, patients must follow the prescribed treatment, increasingly on their own because of success in developing effective treatments that allow ambulatory, self-administered care and in some countries cutbacks in health services that necessitate more self-care. At present, we can help patients stay in care, but we are not so successful in helping them follow our prescriptions closely, dissipating much of the benefit.[29]

Conclusion

Successful bridging of the barriers from evidence to decision making will not ensure that the patient will receive optimal treatment as there are many other factors that might prevail, notably in these days underfunding of health services and maldistribution of resources. Nevertheless, incorporating current best evidence into clinical decisions promises to decrease the traditional delay between evidence generation and application, and to increase the proportion of patients for whom current best treatment is offered. Quick access to accurate summaries of best evidence is rapidly improving at present. Means for creating evidence based clinical policy and applying this policy judiciously and conscientiously are under development, with this final frontier being advanced by current health services and information research.

References

1 Sackett DL, Rosenberg WMC, Gray JAM, Haynes RB. Evidence based medicine: what it is and what it isn't. *BMJ* 1996;**312**:71–2.
2 Mair, F, Crowley T, Bundred P. Prevalence, aetiology, and management of heart failure in general practice, *BJGP* 1996;**46**:77–9.
3 Mashru M, Lant A. Interpractice audit of diagnosis and management of hypertension in primary care: educational intervention and review of medical records. *BMJ* 1997;**314**:942–6.

4 Sudlow M, Rodgers H, Kenny R, Thomson R. Population-based study of use of anticoagulants among patients with atrial fibrillation in the community. *BMJ* 1997;**314**: 1529–30.

5 Antman EM, Lau J, Kupelnick B, Mosteller F, Chalmers TC. A comparison of results of meta-analyses of randomized control trials and recommendations of experts. *JAMA* 1992; **268**:240–8.

6 Michaud C, Murray CJL. Resources for health research and development in 1992: a global overview. Annex 5 in: *Investing in health research and development*. Report of the Ad Hoc Committee on Health Research Relating to Future Intervention Options. Geneva: World Health Organization, 1996.

7 Haynes RB. Loose connections between peer-reviewed clinical journals and clinical practice. *Ann Intern Med* 1990;**113**:724–8.

8 Sackett DL, Richardson SR, Rosenberg W, Haynes RB. *Evidence based medicine: how to practice and teach EBM*. London: Churchill Livingstone, 1997.

9 Haynes RB. The origins and aspirations of *ACP Journal Club* [editorial]. *ACP J Club* 1991; **Jan–Feb**: A18. (*Ann Intern Med* 1991;**114**(1).)

10 Sackett DL, Haynes RB. On the need for evidence based medicine. *Evidence based Med* 1995;**1**:5.

11 *The Cochrane Library*. London: BMJ Publishing Group. Electronic subscription serial.

12 Hersh W. Evidence based medicine and the Internet [editorial]. *ACP J Club* 1996;**125**: A-14.

13 Johnston ME, Langton KB, Haynes RB, Mathieu A. Effects of computer-based clinical decision support systems on clinician performance and patient outcome. A critical appraisal of research. *Ann Intern Med* 1994;**120**:135–42.

14 Gray JAM, Haynes RB, Sackett DL, Cook DJ, Guyatt GH. Transferring evidence from health care research into medical practice: 3. Developing evidence based clinical policy. *Evidence based Med* 1997;**2**:36–8.

15 Krahn M, Naylor CD, Basinski AS, Detsky AS. Comparison of an aggressive (US) and a less aggressive (Canadian) policy for cholesterol screening and treatment. *Ann Intern Med* 1991;**115**:248–55.

16 Carter A. Background to the "guidelines for guidelines" series. *Can Med Assoc J* 1993; **148**:383.

17 Davis DA, Thomson MA, Oxman AD, Haynes RB. Changing physician performance: a systematic review of the effect of educational strategies. *JAMA* 1995;**274**:700–5.

18 Karuza J, Calkins E, Feather J, *et al*. Enhancing physician adoption of practice guidelines. Dissemination of influenza vaccination guideline using a small-group consensus process. *Arch Intern Med* 1995;**155**:625–32.

19 Doorey AJ, Michelson EL, Topol EJ. Thrombolytic therapy of acute myocardial infarction. *JAMA* 1992;**268**:3108–14.

20 Ketley D, Woods KL. Impact of clinical trials on clinical practice: example of thrombolysis for acute myocardial infarction. *Lancet* 1993;**342**:891–4.

21 Grilli R, Lomas J. Evaluating the message: the relationship between compliance rate and the subject of a practice guideline. *Med Care* 1994;**132**:202–13.

22 Aszkenasy OM, Dawson D, Gill M, Haines A, Patterson DLH. Audit of direct access cardiac investigations: experience in an inner London health district. *J Roy Soc Med* 1994; **87**:588–90.

23 Sutton M. Personal paper: how to get the best health outcome for a given amount of money. *BMJ* 1997;**315**:47–9.

24 Pharoah PD, Hollingworth W. Cost-effectiveness of lowering cholesterol concentration with statins in patients with and without pre-existing coronary heart disease: life table method applied to health authority population. *BMJ* 1996;**312**:1443–8.

25 European Carotid Surgery Trialists' Collaborative Group. MRC European Carotid Surgery Trial: interim results for symptomatic patients with severe (70–99%) or with mild (0–29%) carotid stenosis. *Lancet* 1991;**337**:1235–43.

26 Stewart M. Studies of health outcomes and patient-centred communication. In: Stewart M, Brown JB, Weston WW, McWhinney IR, McWilliam CL, Freeman TR. ed. *Patient-centred medicine*. California: Sage Publications, 1995.

27 Stocking B. Implementing the findings of effective care in pregnancy and childbirth. *Milbank Q* 1993;**71**:497 522.

28 Shepperd S, Coulter A, Farmer AU. Using interactive videos in general practice to inform patients about treatment choices. *Fam Pract* 1995;**12**:443–7.

29 Haynes RB, McKibbon KA, Kanani R. Systematic review of randomised controlled trials of the effects on patient adherence and outcomes of interventions to assist patients to follow prescriptions for medications. *The Cochrane Library*. Issue 2. London: BMJ Publishing Group, 1997.

11 Decision support

PAUL TAYLOR AND JEREMY WYATT

Introduction

The history of computers in medicine is a story not just of technological progress but also of changing perceptions of the role and value of computer-based tools. Our ideas about what kind of tool computers are, and of the uses to which they can be put, have changed as the technology has advanced and as our conception of the part they should play in our lives has developed. Computers were first viewed as tools for performing calculations, then for processing information, accessing knowledge and, most recently, facilitating communication. Within each of these paradigms computer systems have been developed to assist in medical work; within each, systems have been developed which are relevant to getting research findings into practice. There are therefore four distinct ways in which computer systems can contribute to the implementation of research findings:

(1) performing calculations using statistical data to be used in computer-based decision support systems
(2) providing tools which generate patient-specific advice from evidence based guidelines
(3) enabling the development of large, accessible databases of clinical research findings
(4) using computer-based communication networks to make clinical expertise in centres of research accessible to larger numbers of medical practitioners.

The focus for this chapter is systems developed with the specific aim of assisting with clinical decisions. We will consider these under two headings: the use of evidence in clinical decision support systems and the use of computerised decision aids in evidence based practice. These headings refer to categories that overlap but correspond roughly to the first two of the above points. The third and fourth points refer to kinds of system which are perhaps outside the scope of this chapter; for example, CD-ROM as a medium for the distribution of MEDLINE, making the Cochrane Collaboration's work available via the Internet, or setting up telemedicine links to connect GPs with hospital specialists. The role of research databases,

Internet-based resources, and telemedicine services in supporting the dissemination of research findings must not, however, be ignored and will doubtless become an important part of the infrastructure within which evidence based guidelines are developed and disseminated.

First, we explain the concept of decision support systems.

Clinical decision support systems

Modern medicine is an information management nightmare. It is estimated that to practise medicine an experienced doctor uses about two million pieces of information,[1] while keeping up to date requires staying abreast of a literature in which a new paper is published roughly every 15 seconds (see Chapter 1). Clearly, most of the time, clinicians are practising on the basis of, at best, partial information. Smith, reviewing doctors' information needs, concluded it would be conservative to estimate that at least one question arose in every doctor–patient consultation and noted that most of these questions seemed to go unanswered.[2] Where an answer was sought, the most common course of action is to ask another doctor.[3] The difficulty here is that the doctor being asked the question may not be any more knowledgeable than the doctor seeking an answer. The sources which at the moment are most likely to provide up-to-date and accurate information are, however, too time-consuming and expensive to be used by doctors in the course of their clinical routine: a recent British study of medical library use found that only 13% of clinicians' requests and searches were carried out solely for patient care.[4] Clinical decision support systems have been developed in an attempt to make available to clinicians, in time to influence decisions, small amounts of knowledge relevant to the patient and the current dilemma. They save the clinician from the need to formulate and carry out a search for medical knowledge, and are usually able not only to provide, but also explain, advice.

A definition of a decision support system

A clinical decision support system (DSS) is a computer system designed to help health professionals make decisions. In a sense *any* system which deals with clinical data or medical knowledge is intended to support decisions. In practice, however, the term DSS is usually taken to apply only to systems, which help clinicians apply knowledge in particular cases. The definition of the term usually excludes electronic textbooks, hypertext, and text databases which require the user to search for information and do not synthesise search results into a report which applies specifically to a particular patient. Also excluded is educational software, which is designed

87

to enhance a clinician's knowledge, not to assist with specific decisions. Finally, because they do not contain medical knowledge or give advice, computer systems which acquire, process, or communicate patient data are also excluded.

Decision support systems, also called decision aids, consist of a store of medical knowledge, or knowledge base, and a "reasoner" – a computer program which uses patient data to select, display, or apply relevant facts

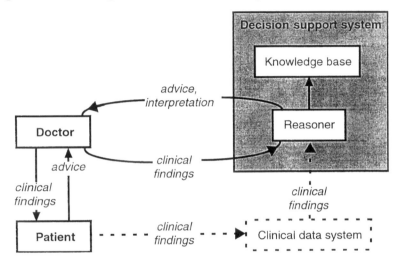

Figure 11.1 Decision support system showing entry of clinical findings by a doctor or via a clinical data system.

from this knowledge store (Figure 11.1). To obtain advice or information from a DSS, it must be provided with patient data such as the age, clinical findings, diagnosis, current medication, test results, etc. Such data may be entered directly by the clinician or obtained from a clinical data system.

The term "decision support system" reflects an evolution in thinking about the possible role for computers in decision making, so that they are viewed as having a supporting role: they aim to improve human decision making without replacing human judgement. Their role is analogous to that of an assistant who, given patient data, finds the relevant pages in a textbook (the printed counterpart of the knowledge base) and highlights only the material which applies to this patient on this occasion.

Kinds of decision support system

Early examples of DSS were developed to help in the diagnosis of patients with acute abdominal pain[5] or in the selection of appropriate antibiotic therapies.[6] More recently, systems have been developed to assist in the diagnosis of congenital heart problems,[7] GP prescribing,[8] the interpretation of ECG signals[9] and radiological investigations,[10] and to assess prognosis in intensive care units.[11] The range and variety of work in clinical DSS is now such that it would be inappropriate to attempt a complete summary here; interested readers are referred to several excellent reviews of the subject.[12-16]

It may be useful, however, to provide a short explanation of the differences between the various kinds of DSS. Systems have been developed using many different techniques for representing medical knowledge, each of which is associated with an appropriate reasoning method. The most

Table 11.1 Knowledge base contents, origin, and reasoning method for common kinds of clinical decision support system

Kind of decision support system (synonym)	Knowledge base contents	Knowledge base origin	Role of research findings	Reasoning method
Bayesian model (causal probabilistic network, influence diagram)	Prior and conditional probabilities; graph representing causal model	Training data; human expert's causal model	Training data can be rigorously acquired; causal model based on published evidence	Bayesian probability calculations
Clinical algorithm, prognostic rule	Coefficients of formulae	Training data	Training data can be rigorously acquired	Logistic regression, recursive partitioning
Neural network (connectionist model, artificial neural net)	Node thresholds, strengths of links between nodes	Training data	Training data can be rigorously acquired	"Black box" variant of standard statistical methods
Reminder or alerting system (protocol-directed care system)	Discrete IF ... THEN rules	Practice guideline, human expert, or committee	Guidelines, authors can base their work on clinical evidence	Conventional programming techniques
Knowledge-based system (expert system)	Interacting facts, rules, semantic networks, frames, uncertainty metrics	Human experts; rules "induced" from training examples	Evidence based knowledge base development	Logic, artificial intelligence techniques

common approaches are summarised in Table 11.1. They can be divided into two broad categories: systems in which medical knowledge is represented explicitly (knowledge-based systems, reminder systems) and systems which "learn" their own rules, whether these are explicit or not, when "trained" on large numbers of clinical cases. In practice, this distinction is not entirely clear-cut since in some systems learning is restricted to assigning different weights to coefficients in a model which is an explicit representation of the problem the system is designed to address. One such technique uses a model that takes the form of a network which represents the links between the different pieces of evidence and the decision options they would support. The process by which the impact of evidence is propagated through the network is known as Bayesian updating, and it is underpinned by the same mathematical theory as the work on decision analysis, described in Chapter 12.

The best known review of the literature identified 793 citations to work in computer-based clinical decision support.[17] Of these, 28 referred to controlled trials. The authors found that 15 out of 24 studies that assessed clinician performance showed improvements due to DSS. Three out of 10 studies that assessed patient outcomes reported significant improvements. This review has since been updated and 53 randomised controlled trials were identified in searches covering the period from 1974 to January 1997.[18] Physician performance was assessed in 49 studies, of which 31 (63%) showed an improvement. Patient outcomes were assessed in 16, of which

Table 11.2 Changes in physician performance due to the use of computerised DSS[18]

Behaviour	Total no. of studies	Studies showing improvement
Drug dosing	9	6 (66%)
Diagnosis	6	1 (17%)
Preventive care	17	11 (65%)
Active clinical care	17	13 (77%)

four (25%) showed benefit. As the figures in Table 11.2 make clear, this review shows that DSS have been much less successful at improving diagnosis than, for example, drug dosing or active clinical care.

It seems clear that decision support systems can improve clinical performance and patient outcome. Equally, it is apparent that many projects end in failure. Despite the enormous energy that has been devoted to these systems for over 30 years, a recent survey was able to identify only 20 systems in regular use.[19] Many of the leaders in the field have discussed the causes of this failure and proposed a variety of explanations, predictions, and prescriptions.[12,19-22] Two of the arguments which have been advanced will be picked up in the next two sections: first, that greater attention should be paid to validating the knowledge bases used in decision support and second, that the use of guidelines and protocols to direct care may provide the most appropriate application for DSS.

The use of evidence in DSS

The only basis for the advice given by a clinical decision support system is the computerised knowledge store. Constructing this involves ascertaining and representing the appropriate set of facts. The process can start by extracting facts from the literature, eliciting them from experts, or collecting and analysing clinical data. The original impetus for much of the work in clinical DSS came from artificial intelligence, where the aim was to represent the wisdom of an expert or a group of experts. The nature of this paradigm – the "expert system" – has changed, largely through the observation that systems must be designed to work in collaboration with the decision maker rather than behave like a Greek oracle which elicits information and responds with a preferred solution.[23] The idea that eliciting information from an experienced physician is an acceptable source for a knowledge base has also been questioned,[20] but the practice is still widespread.

Eliciting knowledge from experts proved a time-consuming task for the expert system designer, and one with which experts were often reluctant to cooperate.[24] It was therefore not uncommon for artificial intelligence researchers to extract knowledge from review articles and books. This practice is not without its difficulties: extracting facts in this way involves separating them from their context and so may render them ambiguous or seemingly perverse. Authors of review articles may attempt a comprehensive coverage of a domain which leads them to include information a general clinician would regard as obscure and irrelevant. Authors may also be out of date: Antman *et al.* discovered that the routine use of streptokinase in myocardial infarction began to be advised in textbooks and review articles only in 1987, 13 years after a meta-analysis of clinical trials would have revealed clear and compelling evidence to support its use.[25] The system designer may be unaware if statements in the literature are controversial or if the terminology used is not universally understood.[26] Van der Lei has suggested that a growing concern in decision support systems is to model medical knowledge as it emerges from research.[21] He cites two examples of systems that are built out of the medical literature, the Roundsman system which models clinical trials[27] and the QMR system[28] which incorporates references to the articles – which are not in this case necessarily systematic reviews – from which the knowledge was drawn.

Friedman and Wyatt point out that the knowledge in decision support systems has rarely been based explicitly on research findings.[29] One notable exception is that of PREOP, a program to help the preoperative work-up of high-risk patients.[30] PREOP elicits input from the user – an internal medical trainee – about the patient and gives advice about drugs and anaesthetic interactions as well as an indication of cardiac risk. The knowledge base consists of facts systematically extracted from journal articles and books, abstracts of which are available in the system. The authors attempted to practise evidenced-based knowledge base development, but admit to having had to balance rigour with feasibility. This means that they were obliged to include facts based on lower grade

Table 11.3 Criteria used to grade evidence in PREOP[30]

For studies of treatment, prevention, or rehabilitation

I   (a) random assignment
     (b) control group
     (c) 80% follow-up
     (d) demonstration of a statistically significant difference in at least one important clinical outcome (for example, survival or major morbidity) OR lack of demonstration of a statistically significant difference in an important outcome where power exceeds 80% to detect a clinically important difference

II   Ia but missing any or all of Ib, Ic, or Id
III Non-randomised trial with contemporaneous controls selected by a systematic method
IV Case series with historical or literature controls OR before–after studies OR case series without controls (each should have 10 patients or more)
V   Case report (<10 patients)
VI Non-clinical study (animal or laboratory tissues, etc.)
VII None of above (author's unreferenced opinion, experience)

evidence. The criteria used to grade evidence are given in Table 11.3. Each fact is graded by the strength of evidence, and the best available evidence is presented first.

As an alternative to basing the knowledge in a DSS on findings in the literature or the opinions of experts, the knowledge can be obtained through research specifically to establish the DSS. The de Dombal system for the differential diagnosis of acute abdominal pain was based on patient data, acquired over many years, which was used to calculate the specificity, sensitivity, and prevalence of different signs and symptoms. These were then used to compute the most likely diagnosis from information entered about a new patient.[31] This relatively simple system assumed mutual exclusivity of diagnoses and conditional independence of findings. In more recent systems the dependencies between different factors are represented in a network and values of the probability associated with a link are obtained from experts' subjective judgements and then revised in the light of experimental evidence (for example, references 7, 32). In a relatively rare example of a system based closely on research findings, Vadher *et al.* have developed a DSS for the control of oral anticoagulants using an empirically validated pharmacokinetic and pharmacodynamic model of the time course of warfarin action.[33]

Designers of those DSS which have not used knowledge derived directly from evidence have attempted to provide a basis in evidence for their work through empirical evaluations of their systems. Such evaluations can include an attempt to validate the contents of the knowledge base. The methodological issues involved in such studies have become an increasing preoccupation in the field.[29] One of the difficulties in developing decision aids which could pass a rigorous validation is in ensuring that the knowledge base includes a complete representation of the domain for which the system is intended to provide support. One response to this problem is to develop systems which, rather than attempting to provide all the relevant knowledge concerning a problem, simply contain a representation of the relevant set of published guidelines. In effect, the system developer places the responsibility for knowledge base content onto the guideline authors. Such systems are described below.

The use of DSS in evidence based practice

It has been argued that the emergence of protocol-based care provides the first real opportunity to use knowledge-based systems in mainstream clinical care.[34] Since protocols oblige clinicians to formalise medical practice they provide an appropriate vehicle for the development of computer aids based on representations of medical knowledge. Certainly, recent conferences on the applications of computers in medicine have included a great many papers on the topic (see, for example, references 35–40).

To date, the majority of computerised decision support tools for protocol-based care have been developed for consensus guidelines. *Effective Health Care* – described in more detail in Chapter 4 – looked at the evidence on implementing such guidelines.[41] The breakdown of the results is given in

Table 11.4 Results of randomised controlled trials of the use of computer-generated reminders[41]

	Studies of clinical care	Studies of preventive care
Measures of process	9/9 detected improvement	11/12 detected improvement
Measures of outcome	3/5 detected improvement	1/1 detected improvement

Table 11.4, but overall they found that improvements were detected in 20 out of 21 studies of the effects on process of care, while four out of six studies of outcome showed an improvement with the use of computer-generated reminders.

More recently, Safran *et al.* described a controlled prospective trial of a computer-based patient record system which generated messages to alert clinicians to events specified in practice guidelines for HIV care.[42] They found greatly reduced response times. Pestonik *et al.* carried out a careful study of the use of DSS with local clinician-derived guidelines for antibiotic therapy.[43] They found antibiotic use was improved, costs were reduced, and the emergence of antibiotic-resistant pathogens was stabilised.

These systems are based on relatively simple guidelines. The decision support requires little knowledge, hardly any patient data, and almost no reasoning. A number of groups are currently working on the development of formalisms, which allow the succinct representation of more complex protocols. Musen and colleagues have, over the last 10 years, developed a suite of knowledge acquisition tools, which they have applied to the task of providing protocol-based decision support.[38,44,45] Fox et al. have developed a language which allows protocols to be defined in terms of a small set of generic entities (tasks, actions, plans, decisions, enquiries) and a graphical editor which allows clinicians rapidly to specify a protocol in terms which can be translated into a computerised representation.[46] An example of

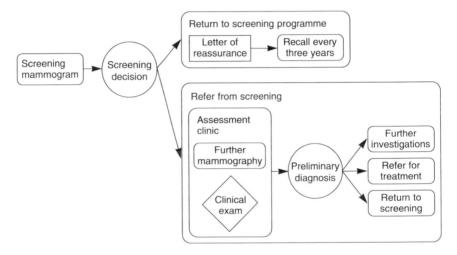

Figure 11.2 An example of a protocol fragment represented in the ProForma formalism, as described by Fox (1997).[46] Actions are represented by rectangles with square corners, decisions by circles, and enquiries by diamonds. Rectangles with rounded corners represent plans, which are composed of sequences of plans, decisions, actions, and enquiries. The arrows are used to indicate constraints on the order in which tasks must be performed. The protocol shown is that used in a computerised decision aid for mammography screening.[47]

ProForma's graphical notation is shown in Figure 11.2. Once the technology has been developed which will allow these kinds of tools to be used to provide large numbers of guidelines within the electronic patient record systems used by general practitioners or to support the management of multi-centre clinical trials, the potential for the use of decision support in routine medicine will increase dramatically.[48]

The further development of evidence based practice will result in the increasing use of guidelines and protocols based on sound evidence. This will be facilitated by, and provide an application for, knowledge-based decision support. The role of DSS in the evidence based practice movement is not, however, restricted to systems which aim to assist in the management of guideline-directed care. DSS are also being developed to assist in the design of randomised controlled trials[49] and advise on the eligibility of patients for such trials.[50]

Conclusion

Thirty years of research into decision support systems has led to the publication of thousands of papers reporting apparently successful implementations. Relatively few of these papers, however, are rigorous studies. The 793 citations identified by Johnston et al. included only 28 controlled trials, of which 21 were, to some degree, methodologically flawed.[17] Clearly, there is considerable scope for system developers to work with health services researchers in the evaluation of decision support technology. Nevertheless, 18 out of the 28 trials demonstrated clear benefits from the use of these systems. The field has, in spite of this, had relatively little impact on clinical practice. For some the lack of diffusion of these tools is due to resistance by medical professionals, for others the tools fail to capture the essence of human practice. Both tools and practice develop together and transform each other.

Proponents of evidence based practice argue for an increased formalisation of medicine and the adoption of formal skills and tools to guide clinical practice. Inserting a formal tool such as a computer system or a protocol into a clinical setting inevitably alters the setting, through the installation or reinforcement of bureaucratic hierarchies, increased structuring of medical personnel's work (for example, through the use of standard data collection forms), and a concentration on data items which can be gathered reliably and unequivocally (to the exclusion of useful but unstructured information, such as details of patient's home life). We need, therefore, to understand the consequences of adopting a tool in a particular setting.

Berg argues that we need to step outside the discipline of the system designer and understand the social, material, and organisational aspects of medical work.[51] The process of designing a tool is not one of shaping it to fit a pre-existing niche; it also involves constructing a niche. Poor design and a failure to consider the practicalities of clinical settings have perhaps hindered the take-up of decision support systems, but such systems could never be designed to fit seamlessly into existing ways of working since the use of formal tools inevitably changes medical practice. And they do so in ways which have drawbacks. as well as benefits. The challenge, as stated by Berg, is to search for ways in which decision support systems can become "familiar yet never totally transparent, powerful yet fragile agents of change".

It seems likely that DSS will provide not just an effective technology to facilitate the implementation of research findings but may also help us to understand how some of the barriers to the implementation of research findings may be overcome.

References

1 Wyatt J. Use and sources of medical knowledge. *Lancet* 1991;**338**:1368–73.
2 Smith R. What clinical information do doctors need? *BMJ* 1996;**313**:1062–8.
3 Covell D, Uman G, Manning P. Information needs of office practice: are they being met? *Ann Intern Med* 1985;**103**:596–9.
4 Urquart C, Hepworth J. The value of information supplied to clinicians by health libraries: devising an outcomes-based assessment of the contribution of libraries to clinical decision making. *Health Libr Rev* 1995;**12**:201–15.
5 De Dombal FT, Leaper DJ, Staniland JR, *et al.* Computer-aided diagnosis of acute abdominal pain. *BMJ* 1972;**2**:9–13.
6 Shortliffe E. *Computer-based medical consultations: MYCIN.* Artificial Intelligence Series. New York: Elsevier Computer Science Library, 1976.
7 Franklin RC, Spiegelhalter DJ, Macartney FJ, Bull K. Evaluation of a diagnostic algorithm for heart disease in neonates. *BMJ* 1991;**302**:935–9.
8 Walton RT, Gierl C, Yudkin P, *et al.* Evaluation of computer support for prescribing (CAPSULE) using simulated cases. *BMJ* 1997;**315**:791–5.
9 Wyatt J. Promoting routine use of medical knowledge systems: lessons from computerised ECG interpreters. In: Barahona P, Christensen JP. ed. *Knowledge and decisions in health telematics.* Amsterdam: IOS Press, 1994.
10 Taylor P. Computer aids for decision making in diagnostic radiology. *Br J Radiol* 1995; **68**:945–57.
11 Knaus WA, Wagner DP, Lynn J. Short-term mortality predictions for critically ill, hospitalised adults: science and ethics. *Science* 1991;**254**:389–94.
12 Shortliffe E. Clinical decision support systems. In: Shortliffe E, Perreault LE. ed. *Medical informatics.* Reading, Massachusetts: Addison-Wesley, 1991.
13 Miller RA. Medical diagnostic decision support systems – past, present, and future. *J Am Med Inform Assoc* 1994;**1**:8–27.
14 Clayton PD, Hripcsak G. Decision support in healthcare. *Int J Bio-med Comp* 1995;**39**: 59–66.
15 Van Bemmel JH. ed. *Handbook of Medical Informatics.* Heidelberg: Springer-Verlag, 1997.
16 Coiera E. *A Guide to medical informatics, the Internet, and telemedicine.* London: Chapman and Hall, 1997.
17 Johnston ME, Langton KB, Hayes B, Mathieu A. Effects of computer-based clinical decision support systems on clinician performance and patient outcome. *Ann Intern Med* 1994;**120**:135–42.
18 Hunt DL, Haynes RB, Smith K. Effects of computer-based clinical decision support systems on physician performance and patient outcomes: a systematic review. *JAMA* In press.
19 Coiera E. Question the assumptions. In: Barahona P, Christensen JP. ed. *Knowledge and decisions in health telematics.* Amsterdam: IOS Press, 1994.
20 Heathfield H, Wyatt J. Philosophies for the design and development of clinical decision support systems. *Methods Inform Med* 1993;**32**:1–9.
21 Van der Lei J. Computer-based decision support: the unfulfilled promise. In: Barahona P, Christensen JP. ed. *Knowledge and decisions in health telematics.* Amsterdam: IOS Press, 1994.
22 De Dombal FT. Assigning value to clinical information – a major limiting factor in the implementation of decision support systems. *Methods Inform Med* 1996;**35**:1–4.
23 Miller RA, Masarie FE. The demise of the Greek oracle model for medical diagnostic systems. *Methods Inform Med* 1990;**29**:1–3.

24 Greenwell M. *Knowledge engineering for expert systems*. Chichester: Ellis Horwood, 1988.
25 Antman E, Lau J, Kupelnick B, *et al*. A comparison of the results of meta-analysis of randomised controlled trials and recommendations of clinical experts. *JAMA* 1992;**268**: 240–8.
26 Taylor P. *Computer-aided decision making for image understanding in medicine*. PhD Thesis, University of London, 1998.
27 Rennels GD. A computational model of reasoning from the clinical literature. In: Reichertz PL, Lindberg AB. ed. *Lecture notes in medical informatics 32*. Berlin: Springer Verlag, 1987.
28 Miller RA, Pople HE, Myers JD. Internist-1: an experimental computer-based diagnostic consultant for general internal medicine. *New Engl J Med* 1982;**307**:468–76.
29 Friedman CP, Wyatt JC. *Evaluation methods in medical informatics*. New York: Springer Verlag, 1997.
30 Holbrook A; Langton K, Haynes RB, *et al*. PREOP: development of an evidence based expert system to assist with pre-operative assessments. In: Clayton P. ed. *Proceedings of the 15th Symposium on Computer Applications in Medical Care*. New York: McGraw Hill, Inc., 1991.
31 Adams ID, Chan M, Clifford PC, *et al*. Computer-aided diagnosis of acute abdominal pain: a multi-centre study. *BMJ* 1986;**293**:800–4.
32 Sucar LE, Gillies DF, Gillies DA. Handling uncertainty in knowledge-based computer vision. In: *Lecture notes in computer science 548*. Berlin: Springer Verlag 1991.
33 Vadher B, Patterson DLH, Leaning M. Evaluation of a decision support system for initiation and control of oral anticoagulation in a randomised trial. *BMJ* 1997;**314**:1252–6.
34 Durinck J. The role of knowledge-based systems in clinical practice. In: Barahona P, Christensen JP. ed. *Knowledge and decisions in health telematics*. Amsterdam IOS Press 1994.
35 Fridsma DB, Gennari JH, Musen MA. Making generic guidelines site specific. In: *Proceedings of the Annual Symposium of Computer Applications in Medical Care*. American Medical Information Association, 1996.
36 Lee W, Kaiser GE, Clayton PD, Sherman EH. OzCare: a workflow automation system for care plans. In: *Proceedings of the Annual Symposium of Computer Applications in Medical Care*. American Medical Informatics Association, 1996.
37 Shahar Y, Miksch S, Johnson P. An intention-based language for representing clinical guidelines. In: *Proceedings of the Annual Symposium of Computer Applications in Medical Care*. American Medical Informatics Association, 1996.
38 Tu SW, Musen MA. The EON model of intervention protocols and guidelines. In: *Proceedings of the Annual Symposium of Computer Applications in Medical Care*. American Medical Informatics Association, 1996.
39 Wagner MW, Overhage M, Rodriguez E, Cooper GF. Representing CARE rules in a decision-theoretic formalism. In: *Proceedings of the Annual Symposium of Computer Applications in Medical Care*. American Medical Informatics Association, 1996.
40 Zielstorff RD, Barnett GO, Fitzmaurice JB, *et al*. A decision support system for prevention and treatment of pressure ulcers based on AHCPR guidelines. In: *Proceedings of the Annual Symposium of Computer Applications in Medical Care*. American Medical Informatics Association, 1996.
41 Implementing clinical guidelines. Can guidelines be used to improve clinical practice? *Effective Health Care Bulletin No 8*. Leeds: University of Leeds, 1994.
42 Safran C, Rind DM, Davis RB, *et al*. Guidelines for management of HIV infection with computer-based patient records. *Lancet* 1995;**346**:341–6.
43 Pestotnik SL, Classen DC., Evans RS, Burke JP. Implementing antibiotic practice guidelines through computer-assisted decision support: clinical and financial outcomes. *Ann Intern Med* 1996;**124**:884–90.
44 Musen MA. *Automated generation of model-based knowledge acquisition tools*. London: Pitman, 1989.
45 Tu SW, Eriksson H, Gennari JH, *et al*. Ontology-based configuration of problem-solving methods and generation of knowledge acquisition tools. *Art Intell Med* 1995;**7**:257-89.
46 Fox J, Johns N, Rahmanzadeh A, Thompson R. ProForma: a general technology for clinical decision support systems. *Comp Meth Prog Biomed* 1997;**54**:59-67.

47 Taylor P, Fox J, Todd-Pokropek A. Computer aids for decision making in radiology. In: Lemke HU, Vannier MW, Inamura K, Farman AG. ed. *Computer-assisted radiology.* Amsterdam: Elsevier, 1996.
48 Kalra D. Electronic health records: the European scene. *BMJ* 1994;**309**:1358–63.
49 Wyatt JC, Altman DG, Heathfield HA, Pantin CF. Development of Design-a-Trial, a knowledge-based critiquing system for authors of clinical trial protocols. *Comp Meth Prog Biomed* 1994;**43**:283–91.
50 Carlson RW, Tu SW, Lane NM, *et al.* Computer-based screening of patients with HIV/AIDS for clinical trial eligibility. *On-line J Clin Trials* 1995; Doc. no. 179.
51 Berg M. *Rationalizing medical work.* Cambridge, Massachusetts: MIT Press, 1997.

12 Decision analysis and the implementation of research findings

R J LILFORD, S G PAUKER, DAVID BRAUNHOLTZ, AND JIRI CHARD

Introduction

Evidence based medicine consists of more than just reading the results of research and applying them to patients. This is because patients have particular features which may make them atypical of the "average" patient studied in, for example, a clinical trial.[1] These particularities are of two types:

(1) factors affecting probability, for example, the probability that treatments will have the same (absolute and relative) effects as those measured in the trial
(2) the values (or utilities) which affect how much side-effect a person is prepared to trade off against treatment advantages.

For these reasons, it is necessary to particularise from trial results. This is usually done intuitively but decision analysis provides the intellectual framework for an explicit decision making algorithm, the rigor of which can be subject to criticism and improvement. However, it is currently unrealistic (due to time constraints) to do a decision analysis separately for each patient. In the long term, computer programs may enable us to overcome this problem. In the meantime, decision analyses can be done for categories of patient with similar clinical features and personal utilities. The results of such "generic" decision analyses are a sound basis for guidelines. Decision analysis thus provides a rational *interpretative* function to get from evidence to implementation.

Decision analysis is described in detail elsewhere,[2-5] but essentially it involves constructing a flow diagram or decision tree showing the available choices and their possible consequences. The probabilities of the various outcomes (contingent upon treatment options and antecedent events) are

99

then added to the diagram. Lastly, the value of each outcome – its relative desirability or undesirability – is incorporated as a so-called "utility". Given the flow diagram, the probabilities, and the individual utilities, the "best" treatment can be calculated. This is the treatment which maximises expected utility by taking into account the probabilities of the various outcomes and how these are valued. The numerical calculations (once probabilities and values are known) are very easy. We will explain decision analysis with an example.

An example – how does it work in practice?

Megatrials[6] show that clot-busting drugs save lives in suspected myocardial infarction (MI). However, these drugs can cause stroke which may leave the patient severely incapacitated. Also, there is a choice of drugs – the genetically engineered "accelerated" tissue plasminogen activator (tPA) is more effective in preventing death from heart attack than streptokinase (SK), but it has a higher chance of causing a stroke. The risk of causing a stroke does not depend on when treatment is given. However, the probability of preventing death from heart attack does depend on how soon treatment begins after onset of symptoms and on individual risks. Individual risks depend on the probability that the patient has actually had a heart attack and the risk of death given a heart attack. Further complicating the picture, the relative advantage of tPA over SK in preventing cardiac death dissipates after about six hours, and thrombolytic drugs can cause other complications (haemorrhage and anaphylaxis).

So what do we do about all these factors? Kellett and Clarke[7] did a systematic review and then modelled all these variables by decision analysis. We have distilled the probabilities of the main outcomes in Table 12.1 and reproduced a simplified decision diagram in Figure 12.1. "Specimen" utilities are used for the various outcomes; a value of 1 for healthy survival and 0 for death. About half the victims of stroke in these circumstances will survive, but often with incapacity – the mean utility of post-stroke existence is 0.5.[8] The results of running the base case model (i.e. for a person "typical" of participants in trials of thrombolysis) are shown in Table 12.2. Clearly, there is much expected utility to be gained by giving the clot buster and, moreover, tPA is the drug of choice. Even if we assume a passionate desire to avoid the disability of stroke, giving it a utility of -1 (i.e. a healthy person who would equate a 20% risk of death with a 10% risk of stroke), the above therapies remain optimal (data not shown). However, we get very different results as we move away from the base case. For example, chest pain in a 55-year-old man with a normal ECG is associated with a risk of MI of only 17%, and clot busters stand to lower expected utility in these circumstances. The same man with normal ST

Table 12.1 Probabilities of various events (expressed as percentages) according to therapy, aspirin by itself or with either streptokinase or tPA.

	a (with aspirin)	b (with streptokinase)	c (with tissue plasminogen activator)
P3 = probability of dying of myocardial infarction	11.5	$11.5 \times 0.75 = 8.6$	$8.6 \times 0.8 = 6.9$
P4 = probability of surviving CVA	0.2	0.5	0.7
P5 = probability of dying from CVA	0.2	0.5	0.7
P6 = probability of dying from haemorrhage or anaphylaxis	0	0.2	0.18
P2 = survival without stroke given MI $= 1 - (p3 + p4 + p5 + p6)$	88.1	90.2	91.5
P8 = death from another cause sans MI	2.0	2.0	2.0
P9 = survival from stroke sans MI	0	0.4	0.6
P10 = death from stroke sans MI	0	0.4	0.6
P11 = death from complications sans MI	0	0.08	0.06
P7 = intact	98	97.1	96.74

but an abnormal T-wave on the ECG has about a 24% risk of MI – thrombolysis is advantageous, but only just, and it would be disadvantageous if he was younger (his risk of dying given a MI would drop to 5% at age 45), if presentation was late (after six hours or so), or if the patient was particularly strongly averse to residual morbidity from stroke.

The model presented here is for teaching purposes and it has been simplified accordingly from the original published work (see below), although not as much as clinicians trying to do it all intuitively. Nevertheless, once the relevant spreadsheet has been set up, it is possible to quickly alter probabilities to take additional factors into account. For example, we may wish to consider the adverse effect of clot busters on patients with dissecting aneurysm. We did this by adding an extra percentage risk of death when clot busters are given to people with no MI. This makes little difference to the base case but now makes clot busters the less favoured option in people with lower (25%) prior risk of heart attack, even in the small group where they were otherwise beneficial. Some people may have a higher risk of stroke, say, because of severe hypertension. When this extra risk crosses a "threshold" of fourfold, thrombolysis is no longer the preferred option, even for the base case. We have not taken into account the likelihood that clot busters administered within six hours protect against congestive heart failure (CHF) – reducing this risk from baseline (about 20%) by perhaps four percentage points (life with CHF is valued, on average, at about 0.9). Also, we have treated the problem as having a fixed time horizon, whereas

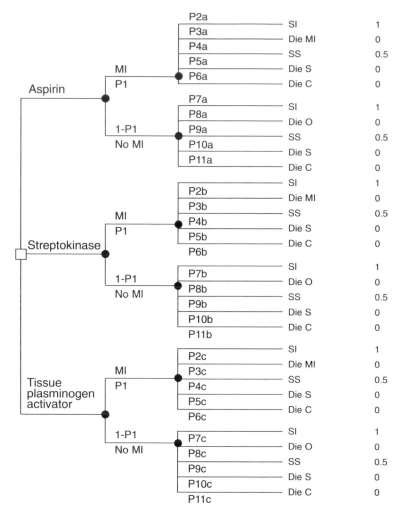

Figure 12.1 Decision tree for the choice of aspirin only versus plus streptokinase versus plus tissue plasminogen activator for the treatment of suspected acute myocardial infarction. The figures on the far right of the diagram are the values. (SI = survive intact; SS = survive stroke; Die S = die of stroke; Die C = die of complications [haemorrhage or anaphalaxis]; Die O = die of another disease masquerading as MI.)

The formulae for expected utilities are:

Aspirin P1{(1*P2a) + (0*P3a) + (0.5*P4a) + (0*P5a) + (0*P6a)} +
(1-P1){(1*P7a) + (0*P8a) + (0.5*P9a) + (0*P10a) + (0*P11a)}

SK P1{(1*P2b) + (0*P3b) + (0.5*P4b) + (0*P5b) + (0*P6b)} +
(1-P1){(1*P7b) + (0*P8b) + (0.5*P9b) + (0*P10b) + (0*P11b)}

tPA P1{(1*P2c) + (0*P3c) + (0.5*P4c) + (O*P5c) + (0*P6c)} +
(1-P1){(1*P7c) + (0*P8c) + (0.5*P9c) + (0*P10c) + (0*P11c)}

Table 12.2 Relative expected utilities (u) of aspirin only (a) versus plus streptokinase (SK) versus plus accelerated tissue plasminogen activator (tPA) given different probabilities of myocardial infarction (MI) and death given MI (all expressed as percentages). (Relative ranking of utilities as in Figure 12.1. The "base case" is highlighted.)

Probability of MI	Probability of death given MI	% improvement with tPA over SK*	% improvement with SK* over a	USK–Ua	UtTPA–Ua	Corollary i.e. Guideline
17	11.5	20	25	−0.00186	−0.00173	At low probabilities of a heart attack, give aspirin only.
17	5.0	20	25	−0.00463	−0.00615	
17	11.5	0	15	−0.00382	−0.0662	
24	11.5	20	25	+0.00017	+0.00152	At moderate probabilities of a heart attack, give clot busters only if presenting in first six hours and if prognosis given MI is in the moderate to severe category (for example over 5%). Use tPA.
24	5.0	20	25	−0.00373	−0.00473	
24	11.5	0	15	−0.00259	−0.00539	
90	**11.5**	**20**	**25**	**+0.01935**	**+0.03207**	At high probabilities of MI, give clot busters and use tPA only if less than six hour history. Even at these high probabilities, the benefits disappear if survival with stroke is given a disutility of −1 and either the prognosis for survival is high (95%) or delay is considerable – data not shown.
90	5.0	20	25	+0.00472	+0.00867	
90	11.5	0	15	+0.00899	−0.00619	

* These figures are dependent on duration of symptoms.
NB. A negative figure indicates that aspirin only is preferable.

103

in reality those with CHF and stroke disability have lower life expectancy than those with uncomplicated MI who in turn have lower life expectancy than survivors of non-MI chest pain. For example, the impact of stroke should include not only a measure of the disutility of each year of disability, but also the reduced expected survival. This can be achieved by calculating and summing expected utilities for each potential remaining year. In other words, a calculation like that in Figure 12.1 is repeated for each future year of life that might be lived. The calculations are different for each year by the probabilities that people in one state (for example, healthy survival following MI) will move to another state (for example, death). This is called a Markov process[9] and can easily be handled on a spreadsheet or specific decision analysis software. In the event, two of these factors (possibility of CHF and flexible time horizon) were taken into account in a masterful decision analysis conducted by Kellett and Clarke's[7] original Decision Analysis, and the decision was not "sensitive" to these factors, i.e. the more comprehensive approach gave similar (albeit intellectually more robust) conclusions.

Decision analysis seems the only way to make sense of the complex world of decisions. However, it raises many interesting issues:

- how may probabilities best be derived from the evidence base?
- how may utilities be measured and whose utilities are used?
- is decision analysis a way of having a debate about general issues in care or is it a way to treat individual patients (or both)?
- how can decision analysis be used to make decisions which affect groups of people?

Probability

Probability lies at the heart of most clinical research; evidence based practice is practice underpinned by evidence about probabilities. Probability is also fundamental to decision analysis. It is therefore important to understand probability in more detail.

Clinicians are most familiar with probability in the form of the predictive value of test results (noting that test is used here to denote any information about a patient, not only results from the laboratory). Take a woman who is pregnant for the first time, whose brother had classic Duchenne dystrophy, diagnosed by elevated creatine kinase (CK) levels, and who died of heart failure. She has no living male relatives on her mother's side of the family, and her mother is also dead. In the absence of any other information and the inability to obtain DNA samples from an affected family member or from her mother, this woman has one chance in three of being a carrier for the disease (this takes account of the fact that a third of all cases of

Duchenne dystrophy are new mutations). Typically, in medicine, we do not have just one piece of information about our patient. For example, in the case of the above patient with a genetic history of muscular dystrophy, we may have a serum CK level. Such additional information seldom discriminates perfectly between affected and unaffected individuals, and such is the case with CK.[10] The literature suggests that 70% of carriers will have elevated serum CK levels. Because the normal range is typically defined as the mean plus or minus two standard deviations, 2.5% of normal women (the upper tail) will have elevated serum levels. A simple method for "updating" probabilities according to test results is shown in Table

Table 12.3 Using Bayes' rule to interpret serum creatine kinase (CK) in a potential Duchenne muscular dystrophy carrier.

Elevated CK				
A	B	C	D	E
Diagnosis	Prior probability	Conditional probability of elevated CK	Product (B × C)	Posterior probability
Carrier	33	70.0	2310.0	93.2%
Not carrier	67	2.5	167.5	6.8%
		Sum =	2477.5	
Normal CK				
A	B	C	D	E
Diagnosis	Prior probability	Conditional probability of normal CK	Product (B × C)	Posterior probability
Carrier	33	30.0	990.0	13.2%
Not carrier	67	97.5	6532.5	86.8%
		Sum =	7522.5	

NB. Upper half of table is for an elevated CK; the lower half is for a normal CK. For each analysis, Column A contains the possible diagnoses, in this case only two, but in general there could be several. Column B contains the prior probability of each diagnosis on a consistent scale (this would be the probability of a woman whose single brother had confirmed Duchenne dystrophy and who had no other known male relatives from her maternal line). Column C contains the conditional probability of the observed result for each diagnosis. Column D contains the product of columns B and C for each diagnosis. Column E contains the revised or posterior probabilities (shown as percentages) and is calculated by dividing each product (in column D) by the sum of the products in column D.

12.3. A simplified form of Bayes' rule applies in situations, such as the one at hand, wherein the test can only be positive or negative and a single state or disease (in this example the carrier state) is either present or absent. The ratio of the probability of the observed CK level if the patient is or is not a carrier is known as the likelihood ratio. Given the prior odds (and recalling that odds are simply a ratio of probabilities) and the likelihood ratio for the observed test result, it is easy to calculate the revised (posterior) odds (and hence probability) that the patient is a carrier simply by multiplying the prior odds by the likelihood ratio. For example, in this case the prior odds are 1:2 and the likelihood ratio for an elevated CK is 70/ 2.5 or 28; thus the posterior odds are 14:1, corresponding to a probability of 93%. Further, as data are typically acquired sequentially, one test after the next, the techniques of probability revision need to be applied in a stepwise fashion, with the posterior probability calculated from one step becoming the prior for the next. Some care is needed where tests are not providing independent information on disease state, as the magnitude of the appropriate (conditional) likelihood ratio of the second test may be much reduced.

Intervention studies (typically clinical trials) provide probabilities on the effects of treatments. These studies can be analysed to give two kinds of probability: conventional and Bayesian. Conventional (frequentist) statistics give "p" values and confidence limits which are based on the probability of seeing the observed (or a more extreme) result, given a true state of the world. This depends on assumptions about the true underlying state of the world. However, decision analysis (and indeed, "bedside" decisions generally) require not the probability of already observed results given some true underlying state of the world, but rather the (posterior) probabilities of particular differences in the effects, given the observed data.[11] Imagine a trial comparing treatments X and Y has measured a 10 percentage point improvement in survival with Y. A patient, who is similar in relevant characteristics to those in the trial, does not want to know that this observed improvement has only a 2.5% chance of occurring, *if* the treatments are equivalent. She needs to know the probability that improvement in survival with treatment Y compared to treatment X really is (say) 10 or more percentage points. Such probabilities – describing beliefs – are known as Bayesian, and their calculation requires that a prior belief (expressed as a probability distribution) be updated according to the research results obtained. An example showing how this works (without going into the mathematics at all) is shown in Figure 12.2. Bayesian statistics give a probability distribution for the true value of a parameter, such as number needed to treat (NNT) – the number of patients who on average would need to receive a treatment in order for one extra patient to benefit. A clear measure of the uncertainty in our knowledge of a parameter provides a rational basis for decision taking.

In our example of heart attack we considered two kinds of patient variable. Firstly, there are variables which affect *absolute* but not *relative* treatment effects. Thus people in the 40–49, 50–59, and 60–69 age bands all receive a 25% improvement in mortality with SK, but the absolute gain is greater in the high-risk older group. The second type of patient variable has an influence on *relative* treatment effects. Thus the duration of symptoms affected the efficiency of SK relative to aspirin so that the improvement in mortality reduces from over 25% at less than three hours to no effect at 24 hours. Of course, if trials were infinitely large then we could look up

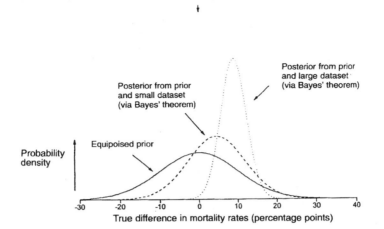

Figure 12.2 The "prior" distribution of probabilities sums up an individual's beliefs prior to seeing new evidence. Suppose a clinician is equipped i.e. has no reason to believe treatment X is superior or inferior to treatment Y, both resulting in a mortality rate around 50%. She believes a difference in (true) mortality rate of up to 10 percent points either way is fairly likely, but that a difference of more than 20 percentage points either way is unlikely. She chooses a normal prior (for convenience – the algebra works out more easily) for the percentage point treatment difference, centred on zero difference, and with a standard deviation (SD) of 10 percentage points. This is actually "equivalent" to the information which would arise from a hypothetical trial with 50 patients and 25 deaths in each arm.

Suppose there is now information from a small trial, with 40 patients in each arm. With treatment Y, 18 patients die, whereas with X, 22 patients die. The observed mortality difference is 10 percentage points. This evidence is combined with the prior belief to produce "posterior" beliefs (which is what her beliefs should now logically be, given the evidence and her prior beliefs). As can be seen above, this posterior is a normal distribution centred a little less than half way between 0 and 10, and with SD somewhat less than that of the prior. The trial evidence has made the clinician's beliefs more precise by adding to her knowledge (reducing the SD), but in fact she remains slightly more influenced by the prior than by the trial. She can calculate posterior probabilities that, for example, treatment Y is superior to X (P=0.73), or that treatment Y is 10 percentage points or more superior to X (P=0.23), etc.

Suppose, on the other hand, there becomes available data from a large trial of 400 patients in each arm, with 180 and 220 patients dying with treatments Y and X respectively. The figure shows that the posterior resulting from combining this with the prior is a much narrower (i.e. more informative) normal distribution centred just below the observed difference of 10 percentage points. Here, the trial is providing a lot more information than the prior. The posterior probability that Y is superior is now 0.996, while the probability that Y is superior by 10 percentage points or more is 0.37.

the precise relative treatment effect for any given category of patient. However, even when overall effects are measured precisely in trials, the effects in sub-groups (strata) are typically imprecise. "What to do" – take the overall effect and apply it to the subgroup or use the imprecise measurement made in the sub-groups? For example, the International Study of Infarct Survival (ISIS-II)[6] trial of clot-busting drugs was analysed in sub-groups. Unsurprisingly, this showed a null effect for people who had had their pain for a long time, but unexpectedly also for those born under the star sign Gemini. On what basis can we "believe" one sub-group analysis and not the other? In a Bayesian sub-group analysis we must give our prior beliefs for how the effect in the sub-group may relate to the effect in the remainder.[12,13] This prior would be that there is little (or no) difference between Geminis and non-Geminis. The observed difference will therefore fail to shift our prior (or shift it very little) and our posterior will remain that Geminis and non-Geminis benefit similarly. Our prior for the difference between patients with prolonged pain and others would (1) be less precise and (2) reflect our belief that those with prolonged pain stand to benefit less than patients with short-duration pain, i.e. from our knowledge of drugs and infarcts, we expect any benefits to be largest if these drugs are administered quickly. In this case the data reinforces our prior belief and enables us to be more precise about how benefit reduces with increasing delay.

Values

The great strength of decision analysis is that it is based not just on probabilities but on how the outcomes are valued. It therefore represents a method for synthesising both the medical facts (probabilities) and the human values which *together* determine the best course of action – that with the maximum expected utility.[14] Decision analysis therefore reconciles "evidence based medicine" with "preference-based medicine".

Of course, there is an issue here about how these values can best be obtained. At heart, values imply a trade-off – the extent which the disadvantages of one outcome can be offset by the advantages of another. For example, survival with radical surgery is higher than with radiotherapy for patients with cancer of the larynx. However, such surgery obviously limits the ability to speak. There is then a trade-off between survival (maximised by surgery) and the ability to communicate (which is retained to a much better degree with radiotherapy). If a patient would run a 10% chance of dying to avoid loss of the power of speech, then she values life with this impediment at 0.9, on a scale from 1.0 (healthy life) to 0 (death). In the example above, the valuation for life impeded by the effect of stroke was 0.5. The subject of the measurement of human values is a huge one which has been reviewed by many authors.[15-19]

Sensitivity analysis, generic decision analysis, and the individual patient

When consulting an individual, it is important to elicit personal values or at least to get a sense of these. However, it is not essential to redo the analysis for every patient in a busy clinic. Decision analysis may also be done outside the consulting room using a selection of different probability and utility figures within a reasonable range – sensitivity analysis. We used this technique to see how the expected utility of clot-busting drugs may vary by medical and psychological characteristics to produce the guidelines in Table 12.2. The sequence of events forming a decision analysis-based guideline and applying it is shown in Figure 12.3.

Often, short-term outcomes are available from clinical trials but long-term outcomes must be derived, as best they can, from observational studies. Since long-term outcomes are often of greatest importance to patient and payer, these should be "modelled" by decision analysis. For example, modelling was required to extrapolate the results of a trial evaluating short-term effects of different types of angioplasty beyond the information collected in the trial itself.[20] Decision analysis is also useful when a clinical problem requires input from more than one set of study results. For example, the effects of hormone replacement therapy have been analysed in many different studies, each concerned with different outcomes and values.[21] Furthermore, observational studies have shown that women have different baseline risks (for example, thin women are at high risk of fractures). Decision analysis has shown how these factors may be integrated to optimise individual therapy.[22]

Decision analysis is used to work out how to maximise an individual's expected utilities. By obtaining median utilities from a large number of people, the methodology can be used to derive expected utilities at the community level. If the costs of various options are included, this is called a cost utility analysis. However, the use of group median utilities creates some thorny ethical issues where, for example, maximising utility and equity conflict.

Decision analysis and resource allocation

Decision analysis can help a patient and their physician decide what treatment to give from within the available range. However, it can be extended to help those who commission services decide which treatments

109

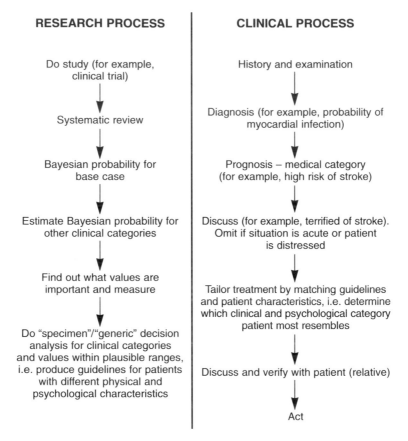

RESEARCH PROCESS

Do study (for example, clinical trial)

↓

Systematic review

↓

Bayesian probability for base case

↓

Estimate Bayesian probability for other clinical categories

↓

Find out what values are important and measure

↓

Do "specimen"/"generic" decision analysis for clinical categories and values within plausible ranges, i.e. produce guidelines for patients with different physical and psychological characteristics

CLINICAL PROCESS

History and examination

↓

Diagnosis (for example, probability of myocardial infection)

↓

Prognosis – medical category (for example, high risk of stroke)

↓

Discuss (for example, terrified of stroke). Omit if situation is acute or patient is distressed

↓

Tailor treatment by matching guidelines and patient characteristics, i.e. determine which clinical and psychological category patient most resembles

↓

Discuss and verify with patient (relative)

↓

Act

Figure 12.3 Idealised scheme showing (1) how the research process should extend to producing probalistic evidence, specimen values, and (on this basis) generic decision analysis (guidelines); (2) how the clinical process "converges" on a particular guideline. If people had more time then decision analysis could be done more precisely for each patient.

should be made available, i.e. to help decisions affecting groups rather than individuals.[18] For example, should insurers, health maintenance organisations, or health authorities fund the availability of tPA (versus SK), or would any marginal money be better spent on another service, say promoting a low salt diet or enhancing an organ transplantation programme. For people, like our patients with MI, the expected gains from tPA versus SK vary from SK better and cheaper, tPA better clinically but the gains are small so it is very bad value for money, to tPA so much better that it is a reasonable buy. When something is better in both clinical and economic terms, that alternative is "dominant". For example, colposcopy is not only safer than repeat smear in cases of mildly abnormal cervical cytology, but it is also probably cheaper, thanks to the high proportion who eventually come to colposcopy either way.[23] Decisions may also be dominant in the sense that both the individual and society as a whole loses. For example, screening for prostate cancer stands to add about six months of life to elderly men. However, the treatment (which will often be administered to men who would otherwise die with, but not from, the disease) has many side-effects whose (dis)utilities have been measured. When these are factored into a decision analysis model, a screening programme stands to subtract four months of quality-adjusted life, despite potential gains in longevity. Clearly, a randomised trial to measure the effects of screening on mortality, with slightly greater precision than has been available hitherto, is unlikely to be a cost-effective investment given current therapy for the presymptomatic disease.[24,25] The situation would be quite different if a less morbid form of therapy, such as brachytherapy, were invoked for screen-positive cases. Of course, the more common, interesting, and problematic situation is where an intervention both increases cost and improves health (for example, quality-adjusted life expectancy). In that situation, one calculates the *marginal cost-effectiveness ratio*, which expresses how much needs to be spent to gain each additional quality-adjusted life year (QALY). This was done elegantly with respect to clot-busting drugs by Kellett and Clarke[7] in their article which we cited above. These ratios can be compared one to another in choosing among strategic uses of the health care "pound". Thus, decision analysis provides the (expected) utilities (QALYs) in cost utility analysis. The values now are not individual values but "average" (preferably median) group values. More detail concerning use of group utilities in decision making are given elsewhere.[26-29]

Decision analysis in research design

This chapter has been concerned with the bridge from research findings to decisions. It is worth pointing out, however, that the bridge can also be crossed in the other direction. Intended decisions or envisaged actions can point to design requirements for research. Thus, in addition to modelling the outputs of research, decision analysis is also crucial at the planning stage.

Decision analysis can inform power calculations.[30-32] By making trade-offs explicit, the size of clinical effect that might be useful to patients and clinicians in their decision making can be calculated. For example the trials of small versus large operations for early breast cancer, even when combined,[33] were too small to show the benefits in mortality that women might wish to trade-off against disfigurement and the other complications of more extensive surgery.[34] A decision-analytic model showed that a proposed randomised trial of antenatal tests of fetal well-being was unlikely to produce clear results – realistic gains were most unlikely to be demonstrated by traditional statistical analysis of a trial because plausible gains were so small in absolute numerical terms.[35] On the other hand, Parsonnet and colleagues[36] showed, by means of a study of the relevant epidemiology and decision analysis, that cost-effective gains were plausible from *H. pylori* screening to prevent stomach cancer, and hence that a trial would be a useful investment. Mason and colleagues showed that the decision to screen for abdominal aortic aneurisms would rationally turn on data within the zone of current uncertainty.[37] Indeed, decision analysis at the design stage may include a monetary dimension. For example, Drummond and colleagues[38] conducted an analysis of the Diabetic Retinopathy Study, a major trial funded by the U.S. National Eye Institute. The trial cost $10.5 million, but estimated savings contingent on the knowledge gained amounted to $2816 million, arising in part from enhanced production resulting from a gain of 279 000 vision years.

In addition to sizing clinical studies and justifying their performance, decision analysis, when applied prospectively to a problem, can help inform which of a multitude of trials should be performed (i.e. where additional, relatively "expensive" data would better inform either health policy or decisions for individual patients).

Conclusion: evidence based care requires a decision analytic framework

Most current research is applied to the production of knowledge, and its use is frequently unsystematic and intuitive. Clinical trials and meta-analyses are carried out with minute attention to detail, then the results are applied in a way which is totally informal, idiosyncratic, and opaque. After slavishly crossing every t and dotting every i, within research protocols competing values are simply "taken into account" when the research is operationalised. If evidence based care is to be seen through to its logical conclusion, and if both empiric evidence and human values are to be incorporated within the decision making process, then (values explicit during the collection of data – implicit during the use of research findings), this duality should be tackled.[39,40]

Building better bridges to get from knowledge to action therefore seems the next logical step for the evidence based movement, and follows rationally from the science of structured reviews and meta-analysis.[16]

References

1 Glasziou PP, Irwig LM. An evidence based approach to individualising treatment. *BMJ* 1995;**311**:1356–9.

2 Keeney RL, Raiffa H. *Decisions with multiple objectives*. London: Wiley, 1976.
3 Weinstein M, Fineberg HV. *Clinical decision analysis*. London: Saunders, 1980.
4 French S. *Readings in decision analysis*. London: Chapman and Hall, 1989.
5 Sox HC, Blatt MA, Higgins MC, Marton KI. *Medical decision making*. Boston: Butterworth-Heinemann, 1988.
6 ISIS-2 collaborative group. Randomised trial of intravenous streptokinase, oral aspirin, both, or neither among 17 187 cases of suspected myocardial infarction: ISIS-2. *Lancet* 1988;**II**(8607):349–60.
7 Kellett J, Clarke J. Comparison of accelerated tissue plasminogen activator with streptokinase for treatment of suspected myocardial infarction. *Medical Decision Making* 1995;**15**:297–310.
8 Tsevat J, Goldman L, Lamas GA. Functional status versus utilities in survivors of myocardial infarction. *Med Care* 1991;**29**:1153–9.
9 Beck R, Salem DN, Estes NAM, Pauker SG. A computer-based Markov decision analysis of the management of symptomatic bifascicular block: the threshold probability for pacing. *J Am Coll Cardiol* 1987;**9**:920–35.
10 Moser H. Duchenne muscular dystrophy: pathogenic aspects and genetic prevention. *Hum Gen* 1984;**66**:17–40.
11 Lilford RJ, Braunholtz D. The statistical basis of public policy: a paradigm shift is overdue. *BMJ* 1996;**313**:603–7.
12 Donner A. A Bayesian approach to the interpretation of sub-group results in clinical trials. *J Chron Dis* 1982;**34**:429–35.
13 Oxman AD, Guyatt GH. A consumer's guide to sub-group analyses. *Ann Intern Med* 1992;**116**:78–84.
14 Swales J. Science in a health service. *Lancet* 1997;**349**:1319–21.
15 Keeney R L. *Value focused thinking: a path to creative decision making*. Boston: Harvard University Press, 1992.
16 Pettiti DB. Meta-analysis, decision analysis, and cost-effectiveness analysis methods for quantitative synthesis in medicine. New York: Oxford University Press, 1994.
17 Thornton J, Lilford RJ, Johnson N. Decision analysis in medicine. *BMJ* 1992;**304**:1099–103.
18 Thornton J, Lilford RJ. Decision analysis for medical managers. *BMJ* 1995;**310**:791–4.
19 McNeil BJ, Weichselbaum R, Pauker SG. Speech and survival: trade-offs between quality and quantity of life in laryngeal cancer. *New Eng J Med* 1981;**305**:982–7.
20 Sculpher M, Michaels J, McKenna M, Minor J. A cost-utility analysis of laser-assisted angioplasty for peripheral arterial occlusions. *Int J Tech Assess Health Care* 1996;**12**:104–25.
21 Johnson N, Lilford RJ, Mayers D, Johnson GG, Johnson JM. Do healthy, asymptomatic, post-menopausal women want routine cyclical hormone replacement? A utility analysis. *J Obs Gyn* 1994;**14**:35–9.
22 Col NF, Eckman MH, Karas RH, *et al*. Patient-specific decisions about hormone replacement therapy in postmenopausal women. *JAMA* 1991;**277**(14):1140–7.
23 Johnson N, Sutton J, Thornton J G, Lilford RJ, Johnson VA, Peel KR. Decision analysis for best management of mildly dyskaryotic smear. *Lancet* 1993;**342**:91–6.
24 Cantor SB, Spann SJ, Volk RJ, Cardenas MP, Warren MM. Prostate cancer screening: a decision analysis. *J Fam Pract* 1995;**41**(1):188–9.
25 Krahn M, Mahoney J, Eckman M, Trachtenberg J, Pauker SG, Detsky AS. Screening for prostatic cancer: a decision-analytic view. *JAMA* 1994;**272**:773–80.
26 Arrow KJ. *Social choice and individual values*. New Haven and London: Yale University Press, 1951.
27 Hudson P, Peel V. Ethical priority setting in the NHS – avoiding playing with numbers. *Br J Health Care Man* 1995;**1**:451–4.
28 Wagstaff A. QALYs and the equity–efficiency trade-off. *J Health Econ*. 1991 V10 p 21–41.
29 Williams A. *Interpersonal comparisons of welfare*. Discussion paper 151. University of York: Centre for Health Economics, 1996.
30 Thompson M. Decision-analytic determination of study size. *Medical Decision Making* 1981;**1**:165–79.
31 Lilford RJ, Johnson N. The alpha and beta errors in randomised trials. *New Engl J Med* 1990;**322**:780–1.

32 Lilford R J, Thornton J. Decision logic in medical practice. *J Roy Coll Phys* 1992;**26**:1–20.
33 Early Breast Cancer Trialists' Collaborative Group. Effects of radiotherapy and surgery in early breast cancer: an overview of randomised trials. *New Eng J Med* 1995;**333**: 1444–55.
34 Lilford RJ. Clinical trial numbers. *Lancet* 1990;**335**:483–4.
35 De Bono M, Fawdry RDS, Lilford RJ. Size of trials for evaluation of antenatal tests of fetal wellbeing in high-risk pregnancy. *J Perinat Med* 1990;**18**:77–87.
36 Parsonnet J, Harris RA, Hack HM, Owens DK. Modelling cost-effectiveness of *Helicobactor pylori* screening to prevent gastric cancer: a mandate for clinical trials. *Lancet* 1996;**348**: 150–4.
37 Mason JM, Wakeman AP, Drummond MF, Crump BJ. Population screening for abdominal aortic aneurysm: do the benefits outweigh the costs? *J Public Health Med* 1993;**15**:2, 154–60.
38 Drummond MF, Davies LM, Ferris FL. Assessing the costs and benefits of medical research: the diabetic retinopathy study. *Soc Sci Med* 1992;**34**:973–81.
39 Dowie J. "Evidence based", "cost-effective", and "preference-driven" medicine: decision analysis-based medical decision making is the prerequisite. *J Health Serv Res Policy* 1996; **1**:2,104–13.
40 Dowie J. The research–practice gap and the role of decision analysis in closing it. *Health Care Analysis* 1996;**4**:5–18.

13 Implementing research findings in developing countries

PAUL GARNER, RAJENDRA KALE,
RUMONA DICKSON, TONY DANS, AND
RODRIGO SALINAS

Developing countries have limited resources, so it is particularly important to invest in health care that works. A growing number of relevant systematic reviews can assist policy makers, clinicians, and users in making sensible and informed decisions. Developing countries have led the way in approaches to ensuring standard professional behaviour through guidelines and essential drug programmes. Reliable research summaries can help ensure practice policies are based on good evidence. This chapter examines the constraints to good practice and identifies opportunities that will help translate research into decisions by professionals and users in developing countries in the coming years.

Introduction

Yakamul, an illiterate villager from Papua New Guinea, was sitting by a fire listening to a health professional from the West tell her to take chloroquine throughout her pregnancy. She retorted: "I ting merisin bilong ol wait man bai bagarapim mi" (translated: "I think this Western medicine could harm me"). She had never attended a workshop in critical appraisal but appreciated medicine could do her more harm than good. She reminds us to ask fundamental questions about the health care we provide, and of our responsibility to interrogate the evidence using scientific methods. It took a few years but eventually we attempted to test her hypothesis.[1]

Removing erroneous opinion from policy and practice is a part of getting research into decision making. Practitioners practise in good faith but, if they are wrong, waste resources and can harm people. Nowhere is this more important than in developing countries where many providers struggle

115

to finance accessible health facilities on a budget of less than £7 per person per year.[2] These countries do not have any slack in the system to waste on a single tablet, injection, or activity that is not effective. Equally important is the time and out-of-pocket costs the patients expend on health care. If, as health professionals, we are providing forms of care that are ineffective, then we are responsible for making their underlying deprivation and poverty worse.

Yet converting research into decisions is not a simple process. Indeed, it is simply impossible when the primary research asks questions that are irrelevant to the study participants. Tropical medicine has a long history of descriptive studies that benefit researchers but do not have direct implications for the participants. For example, a bibliography up to 1977 of research in Papua New Guinea reveals 135 publications describing Melanesian blood groups but only 25 concerned with the treatment of malaria.[3] More recently, researchers have moved to intervention studies that can potentially help the participants. Some quite complex interventions have been tested in randomised controlled trials, such as the effect of improved sexually transmitted disease services on HIV incidence.[4]

Yet even when the research asks questions that can help form decisions, health professionals still confront an ever-increasing pile of medical literature. A good, up-to-date systematic review of randomised controlled trials could have helped the health professional answer Yakamul's question. This illustrates the critical link that systematic reviews often have in getting research into practice. Clinicians, managers, and participants can draw on them, whether they live in Burkina Faso or the Cayman Islands.[5] Reviews and interventions are internationally relevant, but the interpretation nationally and locally is influenced by the resources available and local circumstances. However, just as it is naive to believe that by themselves systematic reviews will change practice in the West, so too is it in developing countries.

This chapter explores ways to build on existing initiatives to improve clinical and public health practice with reliable research evidence in developing countries. It aims not to be fully comprehensive but to reflect the opinions and experiences of the writers to generate discussion.

Constraints

In theory, well-organised, government-funded health systems in developing countries provide good value for money. The unfortunate truth is that in many countries the systems are inefficient, lack recurrent funds, and employ large numbers of health workers for whom there are no incentives to provide effective care. With systems in such disarray, research-led practice would appear to be irrelevant. However, it is precisely these services that

116

governments and international donors are attempting to improve through targeted, focused activities. The logic seems to be that if you cannot make the system work, simply focus on delivering a single component that saves lives. An example is vitamin A supplementation – the type of intervention a good systematic review shows is effective.[6] New ideas and research emerge, so policy makers add more "bullets" to the package. Over time, this process leads to a comprehensive package that the system was not able to deliver in the first place.

Even some established "magic bullets" have little research evidence that they work. For example, evidence that growth monitoring prevents malnutrition and infant death is weak, yet every day health staff and mothers spend thousands of hours weighing children.[7] Standard guidelines for antenatal care in many countries still aspire to provide up to 14 visits per pregnancy, although a recent trial of reduced visits showed no adverse effects on intermediate pregnancy outcome variables.[8] The implementation of effective interventions should take into consideration the whole system, and prune activities where evidence of impact is weak as well as adding new, evidence based activities.

An even bigger constraint is politics. Government allocations to health care in developing countries may be modest per capita, but the totals are large. As a result, there will always be people with vested interests keen to influence the distribution of funds. Capital investment in new facilities and high technology equipment appeals to politicians and those that vote them in, even when these investments may be the least cost-effective. Corruption and kickbacks create incentives that mitigate against sensible decision making. These problems are universal, but comprehensible evidence of effectiveness could provide some support for those attempting to contradict claims that high technology will cure all.

Outside government, there are further perverse incentives promoting bad practice. Private practitioners sometimes prescribe regimens that are different to, and more expensive than, standard World Health Organization (WHO) guidelines.[9] Knowledge is part of the problem as practitioners in such situations depend on drug representatives for information. Commercial companies have much to gain from promoting drugs, whether they work or not. Because of inadequacies in regulation, these promotional activities often extend beyond ethical limits set by many Western societies. Even worse, at times they may come disguised as a form of continuing medical education. The situation is aggravated by lack of effective policy regarding approval of drugs for marketing. In Pakistan, for example, the lack of any effective legislation means that the authorities register approximately five new pharmaceutical products every day.[10]

Yet ultimately it is the medical profession that is the main constraint to change. One reason is that in many developing countries, self-referral and ownership of equipment or hospital facilities is allowed or even condoned

117

by medical societies and training institutions. This creates a situation of conflicting interest, which may explain the irrational overuse of many diagnostic tests.[11,12] Furthermore, clinicians and public health physicians in many developing countries train in traditional approaches. They base their medical knowledge on foreign (mainly European and US) literature and the opinions of foreign visitors, usually supported by drug companies, who are promoting a new product. However, clinicians believe scientific understanding is essential for designing rational treatment; they are respected if they know about the pathology of disease. Medical freedom is valued, and where possible we should avoid strategies to implement research into practice that are perceived as a threat to this.

Established and new initiatives

Trainers, policy makers, and clinicians have already done a lot to engender a science-led culture in developing countries. The Rockefeller Foundation has supported training of clinicians in critical appraisal for over 15 years, producing clinicians committed to science-based practice in their countries.[13] Developing country practitioners are familiar with practice policies, such as those for pneumonia in children,[14] and guidelines have been in use in Papua New Guinea since 1966.[15] More recently, the methodological tools available for improving validity of these guidelines has increased dramatically. In the Philippines, issues for guideline development were identified, and an approach was proposed that may be used by other developing countries.[16,17] Furthermore, the WHO Essential Drugs Programme has taken a strong international lead in advocating rational prescribing. Together with the International Network for the Rational Use of Drugs, they have disseminated research about effectiveness. In addition, they have encouraged management interventions that promote good prescribing practice.[18,19]

Some national governments are now also taking positive action to introduce research-led practice. The Ministry of Health in Chile is setting up an evidence based health office with support from the European Union. In Palestine, doctors are working with their health minister to establish a national committee on clinical effectiveness. In Thailand, the Ministry of Health and the National Health Services Research Institute are setting up an evidence based practice office to guide their national quality assurance programme (Supachutikul A, personal communication). In South Africa, the Medical Research Council have committed to support the production of systematic reviews and evidence based practice (Volmink J, personal communication). In Zimbabwe and the Republic of South Africa, researchers are working with the governments to test ways of getting research into policy and practice.[20] In the Philippines, the Department of

Health has contributed generously to funding for major projects on evidence based guideline development, particularly to direct its cardiovascular disease prevention programme.[21]

Donors and UN organisations concerned with health have clearly influenced the content and direction of health services in developing countries. They have funded one-off research summaries, such as the comprehensive review of vitamin A supplementation.[6] The World Health Organization has also conducted some important systematic reviews, such as the use of rice-based oral rehydration fluid.[22] Now there is more sustained interest in the production and maintenance of reliable systematic reviews relevant to developing countries. Some are being kept up to date, such as a review of the effectiveness and safety of amodiaquine in treating malaria.[23] The Effective Health Care Project in Developing Countries, supported by the UK government aid programme, aims to produce and maintain over 30 systematic reviews in the next four years as part of the Cochrane Collaboration. Already researchers and clinicians in India, Chile, South Africa, and Zimbabwe are participating in the process.

In 1993, the World Bank constructed the "essential package" of effective health care interventions. They made many assumptions in the estimates of effectiveness, and in the main did not use systematic reviews as there were very few available at that point.[24] In the next few years there will be opportunities to revisit these priorities and to draw on more reliable evidence of effectiveness. Donors are also promoting health sector reform, consisting of substantial institutional change in government health policies. Implementation of reforms is biting hard in a wide variety of developing countries. Although reforms are different in each country,[25] the fact that there is change in progress provides the opportunity for introducing evidence based approaches.

Evidence of effectiveness is interesting users of health care. The Network for the Rational Use of Medication in Pakistan is launching a consumer journal to help develop community pressure against poor pharmaceutical and prescribing practice. In India, inclusion of medical services under the Consumer Protection Act has increased the accountability of doctors and made patients, especially in the urban areas, more aware of their rights as consumers.

Future directions

Given the current momentum, how can we further promote the use of research findings in practice? We began this chapter by pointing out that research summaries are often a necessary prerequisite for an individual attempting to make sense of available evidence that is buried under a mass of conflicting opinion. The next prerequisite is to ensure that people in

119

developing countries have access to up-to-date information (See Box 3.1 p 22). It is important to disseminate to a variety of audiences, including other professionals, the intelligent lay reader, and journalists, but efforts to do so in developing countries require further development and evaluation.

However, many mechanisms to implement good practices are already available and well-rehearsed in developing countries. In some, guidelines and standard treatment manuals are better developed than in the West. These guidelines are likely to become more evidence based over time, as there is little point in effective implementation of ineffective interventions. Reviews of specific interventions to change professional practice, such as that by Haynes *et al.*,[26] will help in ensuring change.

These mechanisms must be integrated into service policy and management as a whole, using a layered approach. For example, in June 1995, a large trial showed that magnesium sulphate was the most effective treatment of eclampsia. At that time, one-third of the world's obstetric practice was using other, less effective therapies.[27] The international layer begins with the World Health Organization, ensuring they include the drug on their essential drugs list. Nationally, ministries should include the drug in their purchasing arrangements, and ensure that their curricula and clinical guidelines are consistent with the best treatment. At a local level, midwives and doctors need to be aware of its value. Quality assurance programmes and less formal clinical monitoring should include eclampsia treatment in their audit cycles.

There are a variety of new initiatives to engage practitioners and policy makers in the process of interpreting and using evidence. Some clinicians are examining variations in practice between themselves, as has been piloted in Thailand and is in progress in Chile (Box 13.1). In the Philippines, an ongoing study is evaluating the use of standardised clinical encounters in evaluating practice variation. Another mechanism being investigated, in the area of reproductive health, is that of asking for comments on how professionals would use the results from a particular systematic review in their practice. If successful, this could be used in other clinical specialties.[28]

Aside from addressing the need for information dissemination, policy makers must also address the hindrances to wider acceptance of evidence and evidence based guidelines. In particular, policies on ethical drug promotion should be drafted and strictly implemented, as well as policies governing "continuing medical education" and ownership of medical equipment.

Professionals are important, but it is the public – irrespective of income or location – who make the ultimate decision whether to avail themselves of our care or advice. Paradoxically, people living in developing countries are sometimes the most critical. Yakamul was from a tribe that was poor: life was full of risks, time was always short. The villagers were not afraid to be selective about the components they valued from both the traditional

120

Box 13.1 Framework developed at the Santiago Seminar for Getting Research into Policy (November 1995)

- **Encourage specialist groups to improve practice**
  - start with one particular group, e.g. obstetrics
- **Identify one to six obstetric specialists**
  - keen to use science to inform practice
- **Identify four areas with good evidence**
  - for example, antibiotics in Caesarian Section; steroids in preterm delivery; Magnesium Sulphate in eclampsia; episiotomy/restricted use
- **Measure practice variation in one to six hospitals**
  - either reported (use vignettes) or actual where possible; own hospital staff conduct survey
- **Seminar**
  - present variations in practice to participating groups; systematic reviews in relevant areas; aim to agree working group set up
- **Guidelines working group established**
  - small working group draws up draft guidelines; circulated for comment; finalised
- **Guidelines implemented**
  - through publication, dissemination, workshops
- **Monitor practice**
  - quality assurance/monitoring systems established within hospitals
- **Modify guidelines**
  - working group develop and modify guidelines

---

and Western health systems.[29] As health professionals, we should remember that the public also needs information about effectiveness. In communicating this, we should be honest, humble, and explicit when there is uncertainty in the available evidence.

Acknowledgements

Rumona Dickson, Rodrigo Salinas, and Paul Garner are part of the Effective Health Care in Developing Countries Project, supported by the Department for International Development (UK) and the European Union Directorate General XII. The views expressed are those of the authors and not necessarily the funding bodies.

References

1 Gulmezoglu AM, Garner P. Interventions to prevent malaria during pregnancy in endemic malarious areas. In: Garner P, Gelband H, Olliaro P, Salinas R, Volmink J, Wilkinson D. ed. *Infectious Diseases Module of The Cochrane Database of Systematic Reviews* [updated 4 March 1997]. Available in The Cochrane Library. Oxford: Update Software, 1997.

2 National Audit Office. *Overseas development administration: health and population overseas aid*. Report by the Comptroller and Auditor General. CH 782 Session 1994–5. London: HMSO, 1995.

3 Hornabrook RW, Skeldon GHF. *A bibliography of medicine and human biology of Papua New Guinea*. Monograph Series No. 5. Goroka: Papua New Guinea Institute of Medical Research, 1977.

4 Grosskurth H, Mosha F, Todd J, Murijarubi E, Klokke A, Zenkoro K, Moyaud P, Changalucha J, Nicoll A, Ka-Gina G. Impact of improved treatment of sexually transmitted diseases on HIV infection in rural Tanzania: randomised controlled trial. *Lancet* 1995; **346**:530–6.

5 Garner P, Kiani A, Salinas R, Zaat J. Effective health care [letter]. *Lancet* 1996;**347**:113.

6 Beaton GH, Martorell R, Aronson KJ, *et al. Effectiveness of vitamin A supplementation in the control of young child morbidity and mortality in developing countries*. ACC/SCN state of the art series, nutrition policy discussion paper no. 13. Toronto: University of Toronto, 1993.

7 Ross DA, Garner P. Growth monitoring [letter]. *Lancet* 1993;**342**:750.

8 Munjanja SP, Lindmark G, Nyström. Randomised controlled trial of reduced visits programme in Harare, Zimbabwe. *Lancet* 1996;**348**:364–9.

9 Uplekar MW, Rangan S. Private doctors and tuberculosis control in India. *Tub Lung Dis* 1993;**74**:332–7.

10 Bhutta TI, Mirza Z, Kiani A. 5.5 new drugs per day! *The Newsletter*. Islamabad: the Association for Rational Use of Medication in Pakistan, 1995;**4**:3.

11 Garner P, Kiani A, Supachutikul A. Diagnostics in developing countries. *BMJ* 1997;**315**: 760–1.

12 Dans AL, Distor CA, Dungog PP, Esmundo MA, Espino FR, Ganzon ER. The conduct of periodic health examinations in Metro Manila. Submitted for publication.

13 Halstead SB, Tugwell P, Bennett K. The international clinical epidemiology network (INCLEN): a progress report. *J Clin Epidemiol* 1991;**44**:579–89.

14 Shann F, Hart K, Thomas D. Acute lower respiratory tract infections in children: possible criteria for selection of patients for antibiotic therapy and hospital admission. *Bull WHO* 1984; **62**: 749–53.

15 Biddulph J. Standard regimens – a personal account of the Papua New Guinea experience. *Trop Doc* 1989;**19**:126–30.

16 Tumanan BA, Dans AL, *et al.* Hypercholesterolemia guidelines development Cycle. *Phil J Cardiol* 1996;**24**(4):147–50.

17 Dans AL, Tumanan B (co-chairs). Multisectoral task force on guidelines for the detection and management of hypercholesterolemia. *Phil J Cardiol* 1996;**24**(4):127–40.

18 Interim Report of the Biennium 1996–1997. *Action programme on essential drugs*. Geneva: World Health Organization, 1997.

19 INRUD News. *Newsletter of the International Network for Rational Use of Drugs*. USA: Arlington, 1997;**7**:1.

20 Effectiveness Network (European Union). *A statement of intent by three projects in the International Cooperation with Developing Countries Programme (Framework 4)*. Brussels: European Union Directorate General XII, 1996.

21 Multisectoral task force on the detection and management of hypertension. Philippine guidelines on the detection and management of hypertension. *Phil J Intern Med* **35**(2): 67–85.

22 Olliaro P, Nevill C, Ringwald P, Mussano P, Garner P, Brasseur P. Systematic review of amodiaquine treatment in uncomplicated malaria. *Lancet* 1996;**348**:1196–201.

23 Gore SM, Fontaine O, Pierce NF. Impact of rice-based oral rehydration solution on stool output and duration of diarrhoea. Meta-analysis of 13 clinical trials. *BMJ* 1992;**304**: 287–91.

24 World Bank. *World Development Report 1993: investing in health*. Washington: Oxford University Press, 1993.
25 Martinez J, Sandiford P, Garner P. International transfers of NHS reforms [letter]. *Lancet* 1994;**344**:956.
26 Haynes RB, McKibbon KA, Kanani R. Interventions to assist patients to follow prescriptions for medications. In: Bero L, Grilli R, Grimshaw J, Oxman A. ed. *Collaboration on Effective Professional Practice Module of The Cochrane Database of Systematic Reviews* [updated 3 March 1997]. Available in The Cochrane Library [database on disk and CD-ROM]. The Cochrane Collaboration, Issue 2. Oxford: Update Software, 1997.
27 Eclampsia Trial Collaborative Group. Which anticonvulsant for women with eclampsia? Evidence from the Collaborative Eclampsia Trial. *Lancet* 1995;**345**:1455–63.
28 *The WHO Reproductive Health Library*. Issue 1. WHO:Geneva, 1997.
29 Welsch R L. The experience of illness among the Ningerum of Papua New Guinea [PhD dissertation]. Washington: University of Washington, 1982. Available through University Microfilms International, Michigan number 3592.

14 Opportunity costs on trial: new options for encouraging implementation of results from economic evaluations

NEIL CRAIG AND MATTHEW SUTTON

Introduction

There are various barriers to the implementation of research findings on the effectiveness of health care interventions (see Chapter 10). Economic evaluation, which relates the costs to the benefits of different interventions, faces similar problems but also appears to face a number of additional challenges. Considerable debate continues within health economics on the fundamentals of analysis.[1-4] Notwithstanding these differences, many have argued for the importance of "standards" in published economic evaluations and progress has recently been made.[5-7] More and better information is available and accessible to a growing number of decision makers and advisors.[7] Yet the evidence suggests that the influence of economics on decision making remains limited despite this progress, the emphasis currently placed on evidence based medicine in general and economic information in particular within the NHS, and the opportunity to act upon this information offered by the reforms of the early 1990s.[8] Even where there are high quality data and belief in the broad principles upon which health economics is based, there seem to be even more difficulties in ensuring implementation of the results than there are with effectiveness studies.[7]

This chapter explores why this may be so and suggests ways in which the issue might be tackled. It highlights the assumptions about priority setting decision making processes that are often implicit in the methods of economic evaluations and discusses the divergence of these assumptions

124

from the context for which the results are intended. It is argued that although the assumptions are valid from a long-term societal perspective, they often cannot be generalised to the short term. Incentives and budget mechanisms need to be manipulated to promote the conditions in which the results of conventional evaluations apply, but such changes are often feasible only in the long term, if at all. As a result, in the short term, the results of economic studies could remain rather peripheral to health care decision making unless novel study designs and methods for analysing secondary data are developed, enabling economic evaluation to reflect more accurately the contexts in which decisions are made.

The basics of economic evaluation

There are a wide range of publications explaining the principles[9,10] and describing the practice[11,12] of economic evaluation. In this chapter it is not intended to rehearse these issues or the rationale for economic evaluation,[13,14] but to consider specifically the important features of economic evaluation which may influence implementation.

It has been shown that following an algorithm based on cost-effectiveness leads to an optimal allocation of resources under a number of conditions

---

Box 14.1   The basic assumptions of cost-effectiveness[5,7]

- The decision maker faces a range of options from which to choose.
- There is a fixed budget.
- The decision maker has a well-defined objective which s/he seeks to maximise.
- Any combination of the options is feasible as long as the total costs do not exceed the budget.
- The costs and benefits of each option are independent of which combination is chosen.
- The options are not repeatable.
- All options are fully divisible, i.e. any proportion of any option can be selected.
- All options exhibit constant returns to scale, i.e. costs and benefits rise proportionately with the level of implementation.

(Box 14.1).[15] While economic evaluation can be applied from a variety of perspectives, including patients, providers, purchasers, government, or society as a whole, the societal perspective is preferred by most economists.[6,16] As such, maximisation of the welfare of society as a whole is the objective assumed to underlie most economic evaluations. The

125

process by which priority-setting decisions are made is often implicitly assumed to be a model of "consumer" choice in which the consumer is the person or organisation responsible for prioritising or choosing between health services. In this model, the role of health economics is to provide information on the costs and benefits of competing uses of health care resources.

It is the scarcity of health care resources which means that choices have to be made between interventions on the basis of their expected benefits and the benefits of alternative uses of those resources (opportunity costs). In other words, the notion of opportunity cost provides the rationale for examining the costs as well as the outcomes of interventions.[13] "Measuring 'costs' along the way ... is only an intermediate step to a comparison of benefits and is of no significance in itself."[17] Opportunity cost is often explained in the context of a fixed budget for a health care service. Within a fixed budget regime, the decision to implement one option implies that an alternative option cannot also be implemented. Thus, each chosen option has a cost since the benefits of the alternative(s) are not chosen. Opportunity cost is defined as the potential benefits from the "next-best alternative".

If we adopt a societal perspective, it is necessary to have information on all potential uses of the resources under study.[3] Since this is not feasible, market prices are proposed as measures of opportunity cost on the assumption that in a perfectly competitive market they represent the value of those resources in their "next-best use". Where health care costs are thought to differ from those which would be generated by a perfectly competitive market, it is recommended that suitable adjustments be made.[6]

We shall return to discuss the issue of cost data in some detail later but note here that one of the "fundamentals of analysis" upon which economists disagree is the *definition* of "benefit", as distinct from the *measurement* of benefits, which also generates heated debate amongst economists. Much of economic theory assumes that benefit, or social welfare, should be defined in terms of the utility or satisfaction that individuals derive from the consumption of goods and services, in this context the receipt of health care. In this so-called "welfarist" approach, social welfare is given by the sum of the utility enjoyed by each individual in society.[18] The source of utility itself generates debate amongst economists, some arguing that utility is derived solely from the impact of health care on states of health, others arguing that the *process* of being screened or treated is itself a source of utility.[19] Information derived from screening tests which may reveal no illness or which may reveal illness without influencing patient management is often cited as an example of process utility.

Others have argued for a less individualistic or extra-welfarist concept of benefit in which decision makers can pursue health and health care objectives which they deem to be in the common good, such as equity, legal restrictions on consumption of drugs or alcohol, or state provision of immunisation, but which may conflict with individual judgements of value.[20] We do not intend to explore this debate in detail but the important points for the current discussion are threefold. Firstly, the benefits measured and the techniques used to do so should be appropriate to the position taken. Secondly, which position is "correct" *is* a matter of debate. Economic evaluations, which are more commonly taken from a welfarist perspective,[21] implying that the benefits of health programmes can be measured by the sum of individual utility, *are* adopting a particular normative or subjective position, with which the decision maker using the results of the analyses might not agree. Thirdly, what economics has to offer is not the correct position in this debate but a systematic way of analysing the costs and benefits of different policy or treatment choices, whatever position is taken. Recognition of these issues is necessary both to understand the ethical implications of the results of economic evaluations, and to help understand why the results generated from one perspective may not be taken on board by decision makers adopting a different perspective.

Whatever the definition of benefit adopted, economic evaluations usually compare programmes on the basis of the ratio of costs to benefits. As Birch and Gafni[2] highlight, this requires full divisibility of programmes and constant returns to scale. In other words, any fraction of each intervention can be adopted and total costs and consequences of each programme are given simply by the product of the cost–consequence ratio and the volume of services delivered. On the cost side, it is popular to assume a long-run societal perspective in which all programmes are divisible and marginal costs equal average costs.[6,22] However, on the benefits side, this would imply that the incremental effectiveness of the programme does not change as a larger number of individuals are treated, which is unlikely if patients are selectively prioritised in terms of likely capacity to benefit from services. In this case, programmes should be compared on the basis of the ratio of additional costs to additional benefits (the incremental cost-effectiveness ratio).[23] However, often it is difficult to compare all feasible options because different comparators are being used for different interventions.[24] In this case, a linear programming approach could be adopted which allows for divisible, partially divisible, and indivisible programmes.[25]

However, while we agree that such an exercise may represent the optimal solution in a "first-best" world, there are a number of institutional reasons why this is unlikely to be optimal in practice. In the next section we describe some of these institutional concerns, their implications for implementation, and the current approach to dealing with them.

The current approach to achieving implementation

Of course, the actual decision making context varies from the model of choice set out in the previous section in important ways. Firstly, in practice the process of prioritisation involves a range of "consumers" in the form of organisations operating at a number of levels. The government defines and influences broad priorities through, *inter alia*, policy statements[26] and executive letters to trust and health authority chief executives and GPs,[27] against which performance is measured through a range of accountability review processes. Health authorities have responsibility for establishing local population priorities. Hospitals shape priorities through capital plans and by moving into new "markets". Health care professionals establish *de facto* priorities through their treatment and referral decisions.

Secondly, each of these "consumers" may not share a common objective. Maximising health outcomes (conventionally defined by economists as the product of the length and quality of life) for the population at large does not appear to be a goal shared by either the health care profession or the public,[28] on whose behalf health authorities purchase services.[29] Studies have also suggested that the value to the public of the same benefits in terms of life years saved adjusted for quality of life differ according to the distribution of the benefits between increased quantity and quality of life and according to the nature of the services, for example, whether they are for chronic or life-threatening conditions. Interventions which prolong life appear to be valued more highly.[30,31] In the Oregon experiment, the prioritisation of interventions on the basis of a crude cost utility ratio gave rise to what were considered to be unacceptable "counter intuitive" priorities in which some interventions for non-acute, non-life-threatening conditions were estimated to be more cost-effective than treatments for acute, life-threatening conditions. The lists were rejigged and, although the criteria on which this was done were not made explicit, it would appear to have been to reflect the higher priority which the decision makers felt should be attached to the latter.[32]

Thirdly, all the groups identified above may not be equally powerful in effecting the choices they wish to make. Arguably, the most powerful consumers are the Department of Health who guide purchaser priorities through the policy and accountability review processes, and health care professionals who have considerable autonomy over how much of what treatment they offer to patients. The British internal market was to change this situation by vesting purchasing power in health authorities and boards who were given responsibility for purchasing services on the public's behalf. In practice, however, health authorities still have an arms-length influence over priorities, more akin to employers who subcontract to firms who produce services for them, giving only broad indications of the proportion of the budget to be spent on different services. The control of the health authority as employer is further undermined, both by the reliance on the subcontractor for information regarding the cost and quality of the services produced and by the vested interests of the subcontractor in the pattern of services delivered. There are a number of such principal–agent relationships involved in the choice process determining health care priorities.[33] Imperfections in these arrangements limit the ability of decision makers to ensure their proposals are implemented.

Whether for these or for other reasons, the uptake of the results of economic evaluations by decision makers in the NHS is developing slowly.[8,34,35] The problems faced in trying to inform priority-setting decisions with the results of economic evaluation were graphically illustrated by the experience of the Oregon state health care commissioners, who tried to rank around 600 so-called treatment–condition pairs (TCPs) in terms of the ratio of cost to benefit, where costs were based on treatment charges.[32] Benefits were measured in terms of the difference in utility, or quality of life, with and without treatment. Utilities were assessed by telephone surveys of the public using rating scales known to underestimate the utility associated with relatively minor adverse health states. Single-cost utility ratios were estimated for broad TCPs including heterogeneous mixes of procedures and patients. Both cost and outcome data in the original list were therefore weak and the list was rejected.

It is unclear, however, whether it was the technical weaknesses or the ethical implications of the rankings which led to their rejection. It is possible that it was both. Clearly, the costs used were not true reflections of opportunity cost. However, as suggested above, the nature of the changes made to subsequent lists suggest that the unacceptability of the rankings *per se* contributed substantially to the rejection of the original list. In short, both data quality in, and the implications of, economic evaluations are likely to influence their uptake by decision makers.

Drummond *et al.*[8] address the former issue, suggesting that evidence from economic evaluations may be better incorporated into practice by improving the standard of the information contained in published studies and by changing incentives so that providers are encouraged to adopt a more societal perspective. Contracting and commissioning, for example, were introduced to create a mechanism whereby public health authorities could allocate resources to providers who became more responsive to patients' needs and demands. The *raison d'être* of the internal market was to create the competitive pressures on providers to respond to the choices of agents without a vested interest in current or indeed in any particular patterns of resource use. A more effective alternative to changing incentives might be direct measures, such as constraining the options available to decision makers by including cost-effectiveness criteria in the licensing of new pharmaceutical products.[36]

However, changing institutions and incentive structures is not a simple task. Evidence from the USA suggests that the problem is not one of whether providers respond to financial pressures and incentives, but of whether economic incentives can be designed which encourage clinically and economically appropriate behaviour, avoiding for example cost shifting, cream skimming, and premature discharge.[37] In the UK, contracting has not had the radical impact envisaged by its founders,[38-41] and conflicts between cost and quality are not easily resolved.[42] A number of weak and in some cases perverse incentives have been identified in the regulatory regime governing the market[43] which have undermined both the flexibility of resources within the health service[8] and, as a result, the power of health authorities to effect change through the market mechanism.

In summary, the current approach seems to be one of changing the problem to fit the solution,[43] of undertaking economic evaluation blind to the conditions in which the results have to be applied. In the next section we discuss some additional reasons for the divergence between the solution and the problem and suggest that the solution is oversimplistic. We concentrate specifically on cost issues.

Cost considerations in practice

The issue of the validity of cost data in practice has been extensively discussed in the literature on standards in economic evaluation.[5,6] These considerations, however, have related to technical aspects of the production of the service in question or variations in the costs of inputs, such as hours of medical time, number of days of in-patient stay, type and dose of medication, etc. Such problems may be adequately addressed using sensitivity analysis.[44] However, there are other potentially more important issues such as whether the units of resources required to produce a given service increase in direct proportion to the number of individuals treated, the extent to which opportunity costs are context-specific, and the extent to which decision makers accept that resources are fixed. We begin by discussing the issue of a "fixed budget".

Context, opportunity cost, and the assumption of a fixed budget

Even though the principle of scarcity may be accepted, the assumption of a universal fixed budget does not necessarily hold because, as Sheldon and Maynard[45] emphasise, negotiation over budgets takes place at many levels, from inter-specialty negotiation within trusts to "bargaining" between public and government through the voting process. Players in these bargaining games are aware of the *elasticity* of solutions and their ability to influence the size of the budget. Some "successes" in securing increases in resources may be high profile, such as additional funds for winter crises, waiting list initiatives, and new service developments. The effect of these successes may be to undermine people's acceptance that resources are fixed. Attempts to apply lower-level constraints did little to convince GPs that their budgets were "fixed".[46] Negotiated agreements regarding levels of funding may be particularly sensitive to evidence of unmet demand from which individuals could clearly benefit.

An analogy can be made with the consumption choices facing parents where "need" may be represented by the number of children in the household.[47] A bundle of commodities will be purchased to maximise the welfare of the household within the budget constraint. With the addition of a further child, the budget constraint would inevitably become tighter, but the additional "needs" of the household are likely to provoke a labour-supply response which will also change the budget constraint.[48] Whilst there is obviously an upper limit on feasible resources (there is a limit to the number of hours an individual can work in a day), budgets can be increased within this limit. In a similar way, a more accurate description of health care constraints might be that they are variable but inelastic. If this is the perception in the general population, it may be accepted that there is a need for accountability and frugality but that resources should be reallocated if budgets become too tight. This may explain the reluctance of the public to comply with prioritisation of activities between competing populations on the basis of cost when there is clear "need" established for both groups.[28]

It may also partially explain why the population's perspective is subordinate to the doctor's duty to their individual patients as framed in the medical profession's own code of ethics.[49] Health care professionals might in principle share the aim of maximising the population's health; the medical profession's own ethical code refers to scarcity and the need to use resources efficiently. However, in practice, the maximisation of health in the area of decision making over which doctors exert control, that is, *their* patients, can conflict with maximisation of the population's health. Rather than prioritising use of a fixed resource, when faced by individual patients, clinicians may feel that managing the system-level resource constraint is not their responsibility.

Wherever the truth lies, it is inevitable that the slackness of constraints will vary enormously within the health care sector. Variations in unused budgets are themselves a source of inefficiency relative to a "first-best" world in which money could be moved freely between budgets. In an ideal world, economic evaluations taken from a societal perspective should not reflect these rigidities. Rather, policy makers should change the budget mechanism to ensure the optimal solution is feasible. However, these budgetary boundaries are a reality of the actual decision making process.

Economic evaluations which rest on the principle of a universal budget constraint binding all decision makers equally may prescribe the optimal allocation but are unlikely to have much real-life validity at the level of individual decision makers.

Budget inflexibility causes variations in the extent to which resources under different budgets are employed and this creates the problem that options compared in economic evaluations are not feasible in practice. However, a second problem relates to the inferences that can be drawn from cost data originating in this "second-best" world. Such measures of resources used in the provision of a service do not provide an accurate measure of the opportunity costs faced by the individual decision maker. In practice, it may not be clear that resources have a foregone next-best use when the redeployment of resources is not feasible. As a consequence, the "prices" which have been attached to those units of resources do not reflect opportunity costs in the eyes of the decision maker. In the absence of perfectly flexible budgets, we may observe resource utilisation which is not optimal in the long-run societal sense, but is "second-best" given the limited range of alternative uses of resources open to the decision maker.

Economies of scale and scope in practice

At the hospital level, it has been observed that costs and the number of people treated do not increase in direct proportion to each other.[50,51] It is likely that this is also true for the delivery of specific services within hospitals. Moreover, learning, which is a clinician/service phenomenon, is a determinant of both outcome and cost.[51-53] On the benefit side, if individuals are prioritised on the basis of capacity to benefit, benefits per patient will decline as more patients are treated. Interdependence between the costs of different programmes (economies of scope) have also been found at the hospital level.[50]

The importance of these issues in different circumstances

We have discussed these potential problems with cost data in abstract terms and of course their importance will depend on the extent to which they occur in practice. Much of the work on evaluating medical interventions from an economic perspective has taken place on pharmaceuticals. These interventions may have quite uniform unit costs and may not become cheaper as more individuals are treated. Moreover, they may be more likely to come from a common budget and it may be possible to switch resources between alternatives quite easily. However, interventions that require capital goods such as equipment become cheaper per person treated as the number of individuals treated expands.

It is perhaps labour inputs which are of particular interest. The amount of resource available is likely to be quite flexible as "effort" can be manipulated and will respond to "demand". Therefore, it is likely that there will be increasing returns to scale in numbers treated although this may be offset by decreasing returns to scale in quality. We may also expect problems in switching these resources across different budget boundaries.

Alternative options for promoting economic considerations in practice

Opportunity costs are context-specific because they are related to the available budget and the range of feasible local alternatives being evaluated.[54] To assess whether estimated costs can be generalised to other contexts it has been proposed that, in addition to an overall cost figure, input requirements for evaluated alternatives be presented in disaggregated form.[6,55] However, this still does not take account of stepped relationships between costs and the number of patients treated.

Therefore, to reflect opportunity cost more accurately, Birch et al.[54] propose a three-stage approach to evaluating proposed changes:

(1) evaluate the expected additional benefits from the proposed change
(2) identify the resources needed and where they are likely to come from
(3) estimate the benefits which would be lost from stopping these activities.

This requires a fundamentally different design to the standard method of allocating equal numbers to different treatments and then counting the costs of production and the benefits. In this section we discuss an alternative method of constructing a trial which implements this framework by holding opportunity costs constant.

These proposed designs are examples of one of the few options proposed by Birch and Gafni[2] for ensuring cost-effectiveness studies are compatible with welfare economics. In these designs the aim is to express opportunity costs in non-monetary terms. The idea of expressing opportunity costs in non-monetary terms is not new. In a series of applications, Torgerson and colleagues have indicated how many more individuals could have received treatment if relatively costly service options were not adopted.[56-58]

Studies of proposed changes to health care delivery include some or all of the following considerations: different interventions (for example, group counselling or individual interviews); different inputs (for example, general practitioners or practice nurses); and/or different populations, perhaps defined on the basis of age groups. To simplify the exposition we consider three possible types of comparisons:

133

(1) a comparison of different interventions delivered by the same inputs to the same population
(2) a comparison of the same intervention delivered by the same inputs on different populations
(3) a comparison of the same intervention delivered by different inputs on the same population.

Different interventions delivered by the same inputs to the same population

The basic approach to comparisons of this type is to allocate equal levels of resources to each programme in the study. Sutton shows how such a cost-constrained design might look in practice by considering a hypothetical example of a brief versus more intensive intervention for alcoholism.[59] This example, which uses effectiveness figures produced by Chapman and Huygens,[60] is reproduced in Table 14.1. Although the brief intervention is

Table 14.1 Hypothetical cost-constrained study of a brief versus more intensive intervention for alcoholism[60,61]

Programme	Staff time (full-time equivalent)	Estimated number of subjects treated	Rate of problem-free drinking (%)[c]	Number of problem-free drinkers
Out-patient	1.5	10[a]	28.6	3
Confrontational interview	1.5	72[b]	22.2	16

[a] Based on twice-weekly sessions for two groups of five subjects run by a multidisciplinary team of three half-time workers over a six-week period.
[b] Based on two-hourly sessions at a rate of one each per day for four days per week by three half-time workers over a six-week period.
[c] Source: Chapman and Huygens.[60]

no more effective per person than the intensive intervention, it produces successful outcomes for many more individuals (16 v 3). Therefore, the opportunity costs of allocating 1.5 full-time equivalent workers to the intensive intervention are readily seen in the outcome figures.

This cost-constrained design has several potentially useful features. Firstly, it more directly relates to the problem of achieving the most health outcome from a fixed budget. Secondly, by comparing alternatives at a given input level, it allows for partial or full indivisibility and increasing or decreasing returns to scale. Of course, the problem of generalisability of a production function from a certain setting remains, as does the possibility of economies of scope. Multi-site studies would help in this regard.[44]

In addition, this approach makes a number of assumptions in making cost-effectiveness ratios rather more explicit. The higher per-person resource

134

requirements of some interventions become apparent because less people can be treated and the trade-off between quantity and quality is no longer hidden in the cost-effectiveness ratio. By specifying the resources used in the cost-constrained design, comparisons across studies are still possible.

The study design is likely to result in different numbers of patients being treated in each arm of the trial. This unequal randomisation will increase the statistical power of the study since more patients are allocated to the less costly intervention.[61] Sutton shows that if ethics are extended to those who miss out on receiving treatment because of the resources used (i.e. those who bear the opportunity cost), there are no additional ethical problems with exposing different numbers of patients *ex ante* to treatments which may be of different effectiveness *ex post*.[59]

A cost-constrained design may also reduce the amount of involvement needed from economists. In some situations it may only be necessary to consider the major components of cost.[6] Evaluations may be able to proceed without detailed cost analysis, even though the resultant analyses would be partial on the cost side. With its provider-based focus, this might encourage clinicians to become involved in economic evaluations.[17]

The same intervention delivered by the same inputs to different populations

Torgerson and colleagues provide examples of this type of comparison.[56–58] Because such comparisons are based on reallocation *within* the relevant budget, they cannot be compared with policy changes involving shifts in resources across budgets. One of the studies considers changing the age group to which breast cancer screening is targeted and indicates greater effectiveness of screening older age groups.[57] Fundamentally, the decision depends on the importance attached to treating different groups of the population.

The same intervention delivered by different inputs to the same population

The third possible comparison is the most difficult to evaluate without recourse to cost information. For example, we may wish to compare the cost-effectiveness of intervention delivered by either a hospital consultant or a general practitioner. The traditional approach would be to value each staff input at its wage rate. This implies an opportunity cost of time equal to the wage rate which is only justifiable in terms of a perfectly competitive labour market.

135

In practice, we would want to identify which activities would be displaced for the GP and taken up by the consultant. The changing demands on the consultant and GP may only provoke corresponding labour-supply responses (i.e. the consultant works slightly less hours and the GP slightly more) or changes in the quality of services for other patients. The problem is essentially that the traditional study design does not fully answer the question since the proposed change of work for the consultant should be evaluated alongside the proposed change of work for the GP. The appropriate design for this type of comparison should be to identify the *full* implications of the proposed change for the *total* benefit produced by those inputs.

Behavioural models of decision making and cost-effectiveness

The approach above replicates the conditions facing a decision maker as well as upholding more rigorously the principles of economic theory. However, though necessary to increase the relevance of economic evaluation to decision makers, it is unlikely to be sufficient. Other factors affect decision makers. Behavioural models of choice are required which explain the decisions made by those in strategic positions. Such models need to address the objectives and values of key decision makers, the incentives they face in choosing between alternatives treatments, and the constraints they face in making free and informed choice. They are required both to increase our understanding of why even good economics information might not be used and to understand the constraints and objectives which we should be trying to incorporate into study designs.

In this section, we discuss two examples of behavioural frameworks which have been developed for explaining clinician behaviour. The first model considers how the notions of benefits and opportunity cost are incorporated into clinicians' decision making behaviour.[63] The second considers the diffusion of information and how individual decisions may be influenced by group behaviour.[64]

Whynes develops a behavioural model of clinicians' decisions to treat in which treatment choice is modelled as a utility function in which the clinician's utility is a function of: net benefit; perceived costs; a "coefficient of diagnostic confidence" dependent on the individual clinician's skills and the individual patient's condition; and the personal interests of clinicians in particular treatment choices.[63] Perceived costs are given by: the subjective probabilities of each possible outcome; the expected cost of each outcome; and the physician's view of the importance of the cost of treatment relative to the benefits.

136

Information on cost-effectiveness would influence the subjective probabilities in this model of the treatment decision. It would not necessarily influence the "coefficient of diagnostic confidence", the importance attached to the opportunity cost of the resources involved, the utility derived by the clinician from different outcomes, nor the incentives faced by the clinician to pursue a particular treatment choice. Whynes concludes that "the acquisition of medical evidence can offer only limited scope for harmonising clinical judgements over the desirability of intervention in specific situation". Information influences subjective probabilities but does not replace or determine them, and nor does it necessarily impact upon the other factors influencing clinician behaviour.

Escarce's model of the factors influencing clinicians' adoption of new treatment technologies hypothesises that factors which increase the revenue, reduce the costs, or reduce the perceived uncertainty associated with a new technology will increase the speed at which it is adopted.[64] The latter factor is crucial since it is a function of both the economic evidence available, and the attitude to risk of potential adopters. Escarce's empirical results show that clinicians form a heterogeneous group of more or less risk-averse potential adopters whose behaviour is influenced by the availability of information and by the adoption of new technology by "product champions". Mimicry of "product champions" may be more efficient than reassessment of the costs and benefits of a particular treatment from the available information.[65] This may suggest that different people respond to different types of information regarding the potential costs and benefits of alternative treatments, some responding to the formal evidence of controlled trials and systematic reviews, others to the experiential evidence of personal or colleagues' use of particular technologies. Hirshleifer's[65] model demonstrates how this type of interdependent behaviour can lead to unstable fads and fashions.

The analysis of health care delivery which reflects opportunity costs and not production costs should be conducted in the context of existing analysis on the economic behaviour of decision makers. Economists have developed a substantial body of theoretical and empirical work explaining, *inter alia*, the impact of health care on health relative to the influence of other factors such as "lifestyle", environment, deprivation, and education, or the factors influencing clinicians' behaviour with respect to levels or combinations of care delivered. However, the evaluation literature has developed almost in isolation from other economic analyses of health and health care. For example, this wider economic literature would not support the assumptions that one of the main resource inputs to primary care (GP time) is fixed[66] or that slack hospital resources can be easily reallocated.[67]

Therefore, if we cannot identify the alternative use of the resources, or if we want to allow for changes in the overall size of the budget (for example, labour-supply response), slackness in the resource constraint, or a flexible cost–quality relationship, we may need to rely on behavioural models of decision makers and analyses of observational data. Outside of the health field, an experimental approach is relatively alien to economists who rely mainly on analysis of secondary, observational data sources.[68] The problems of confounding have dissuaded many from relying on observational data for estimates of treatment effects, and economic evaluations have been criticised for utilising these data.[69,70] However, there have been considerable recent advances in the methods for controlling for confounding,[71] and discussion of the advantages of the treatment effects which are estimated.[72] Analysis of observational data offers the possibility of investigating effects otherwise not perceptible, such as macro-level effects[73] and unobservable patient benefits.[74] Increased application of these techniques would be a suitable complement to the recent moves towards increasingly pragmatic trials.[70]

Conclusion

Other chapters have presented reasons why variations in clinical practice may be expected because of differences in decision making, risk attitudes, knowledge, etc. All of these problems also beset the implementation of findings from economic analyses. In this chapter, additional problems associated with economics information have been highlighted.

Encouraging implementation of economic findings is not simply a matter of providing more and better-quality economic evidence. The impetus given to the campaign for improved quality in economic evaluations is based on surveys of the demand side of the market, i.e. the users of the results of economic evaluations such as health care purchasers, and seems to ignore the "harder problems of stimulating and conducting such studies".[2] Establishing standards for economic evaluations[6–8] may actually delay implementation if there is reaction from the supply side, such that researchers who are potentially interested in the principles of cost-effectiveness are deterred from becoming involved. There are familiar trade-offs to be made between quantity and quality.

In practice, decision makers may not [think they] face fixed budgets or alternative uses of resources which are perfectly divisible in terms of either costs or benefits. In addition, they may have objectives which are not coincident with the particular social goals specified in economic evaluations. As noted above, in the long term the former could be tackled by increasing the flexibility of budget allocations, the latter by changing the incentive structure. Whilst implementation of service changes preferred from the societal perspective should remain the long-term goal, there are a number of other options for encouraging the use of economic methods in the short term.

138

Evaluating options for health services to reflect opportunity costs requires three basic steps:

(1) estimate the benefits of implementing the proposed programme
(2) identify the resources required to implement the proposed changes and where they are to be obtained from
(3) estimate the loss in benefits from the original source of funds.

The traditional approach of conducting economic evaluations alongside clinical trials risks leaving cost considerations as an afterthought. Considering opportunity costs means maximising the effectiveness of health care services. If the budget for health care is fixed, opportunity cost should be fundamental to evidence based medicine and the design of studies intended to inform it.

In this chapter we have discussed study designs which place the actual opportunity costs faced by decision makers at the centre of the analysis. We have also proposed that analyses should be conducted based on a range of objectives which decision makers may want to maximise. This range of alternatives could be inferred from analysis of actual behaviour or trials based on what we believe are decision makers' objectives. We believe that by focusing more clearly on the nature of the "real-life" decision and the reason *why* cost considerations are pertinent, this approach may encourage greater participation of providers in evaluation and the use of the results of economic evaluation.

Improvement of the information upon which the choices are made is necessary but not sufficient to ensure an effective role for economics in the prioritisation of health care resources. Priority setting is a complex process of choice. Increased understanding is also required of the processes by which choices are made, by whom, to what end, and under what constraints. This research should be prioritised as a way of ensuring greater implementation of economic recommendations and undertaken as part of an incorporation of economic evaluation into a behavioural framework, using pragmatic study designs and observational data where appropriate.

Acknowledgements

We are grateful for the helpful comments of the editors, an anonymous referee, and several colleagues, including Steve Birch, Diane Dawson, Martin Roland, and Trevor Sheldon. Matthew Sutton is funded by the Department of Health through the National Primary Care R&D Centre. The usual disclaimers apply.

139

References

1 Phelps CE, Mushlin AI. On the (near) equivalence of cost-effectiveness and cost–benefit analysis. *Int J Tech Assess Health Care* 1991;7:12–21.

2 Birch S, Gafni A. Cost-effectiveness/utility analyses. Do current decision rules lead us to where we want to be? *J Health Econ* 1992;11:279–96.

3 Pauly MV. Valuing health benefits in money terms. In: Sloan FA. ed. *Valuing health care: costs, benefits, and effectiveness of pharmaceuticals and other medical technologies*. Cambridge, Cambridge University Press, 1995.

4 Garber AM, Phelps CE. Economic foundations of cost-effectiveness analysis. *J Health Econ* 1997;16:1–31.

5 Weinstein MC, Siegel JE, Gold MR, Kamlet MS, Russell LB. Recommendations of the panel on cost-effectiveness in health and medicine, *JAMA* 1996;276(15):1253–8.

6 Drummond MF, Jefferson TO. Guidelines for authors and peer reviewers of economic submissions to the *BMJ*. *BMJ* 1996;313:275–83.

7 Sheldon TA, Vanoli A. Providing research intelligence to the NHS: the role of the NHS Centre for Reviews and Dissemination. In: Towse A. ed. *Guidelines for the economic evaluation of pharmaceuticals: can the UK learn from Australia and Canada?* London: OHE, 1997.

8 Drummond M, Cooke J, Walley T. Economic evaluation under managed competition: evidence from the UK. *Soc Sci Med* 1997;45(4):583–95.

9 Drummond MF, Stoddart GS, Torrance GW. *Methods for the economic evaluation of health care programmes*. Oxford: Oxford University Press, 1987.

10 Sloan FA. ed. *Valuing health care: costs, benefits, and effectiveness of pharmaceuticals and other medical technologies*. Cambridge: Cambridge University Press, 1995.

11 Drummond MF, Mason J. Reporting guidelines for economic studies [editorial]. *Health Econ* 1995;4:85–94.

12 Briggs A, Sculpher M. Sensitivity analysis in economic evaluation: a review of published studies. *Health Econ* 1995;4(5):355–72.

13 Williams A. How should information on cost-effectiveness influence clinical practice? In: Delamothe T. ed. *Outcomes into clinical practice*. London: BMJ Publishing Group, 1994.

14 Williams A. Economics, society, and health care ethics. In: Gillon R. ed. *Principles of health care ethics*. Chichester: Wiley, 1994.

15 Weinstein MC, Zeckhauser R. Critical ratios and efficient allocation. *J Public Econ* 1973; 2:147–57.

16 Johanesson M. A note on the depreciation of the societal perspective in economic evaluation of health care. *Health Policy* 1995;33:59–66.

17 Dowie J. Clinical trials *and* economic evaluations? No, there are only evaluations. *Health Econ* 1997;6:87–9.

18 Mishan EJ. *Cost benefit analysis*. Cambridge, Massachusetts: Unwin Hyman Ltd, 1988.

19 Ryan M, Shackley P. Assessing the benefits of health care: how far should we go? *Qual Health Care* 19XX;4(3):207–13.

20 Sugden R, Williams A. *The principles of practical cost–benefit analysis*. Oxford: Oxford University Press, 1978.

21 Culyer AJ. The normative economics of health care finance and provision. *Ox Rev Econ Policy* 1989;5(1):34–58.

22 Knapp M, Beecham J, Anderson J, *et al.* The TAPS Project. 3: predicting the community costs of closing psychiatric hospitals. *Br J Psychiat*, 1990;157:661–70.

23 Torgerson DJ, Spencer A. Marginal costs and benefits. *BMJ* 1996;312:35–6.

24 Birch S. Gafni A. Cost-effectiveness ratios: in a league of their own. *Health Policy* 1994; 28:133–41.

25 Stinnett AA, Paltiel AD. Mathematical programming for the efficient allocation of health care resources. *J Health Econ* 1996;15:641–53.

26 Scottish Office Home and Health Department. *Scotland's health: a challenge to us all.* Edinburgh: HMSO, 1992.

27 NHS Executive. *Changing the internal market*. EL(97)33. Leeds: Department of Health, 1997.

28 Nord E, Richardson J, Street A, Kuhse H, Singer P. Who cares about cost? Does economic analysis impose or reflect social values? *Health Policy* 1995;**34**:79–94.

29 Lomas J. Reluctant rationers: public input to health care priorities. *J Health Serv Res Policy* 1997;**2**(2):103–11.

30 Abel Olsen J, Donaldson C. Helicopters, hearts, and hips: using willingness to pay to set priorities for public sector health care programmes. *Soc Sci Med* 1998 v 46 p 1–12.

31 Nord E. The trade off between severity of illness and treatment effect in cost–value analysis of health care. *Health Policy* 1993;**24**:227–38.

32 Tengs TO. An evaluation of Oregon's Medicaid rationing algorithms. *Health Econ* 1996; **5**:171–81.

33 Mooney G, Ryan M. Agency in health care – getting beyond first principles, *J Health Econ* 1993;**12**(2):125–35.

34 Ham C. Priority setting in the NHS: reports from six districts. *BMJ* 1993;**307**:435–8.

35 Redmayne S, Klein R. *Small steps, big goals: purchasing policies in the NHS.* Research paper 21. Birmingham: NAHAT, 1996.

36 Drummond MF, Aristides M. The Australian cost-effectiveness guidelines: an update. In: Towse A. ed. *Guidelines for the economic evaluation of pharmaceuticals: can the UK learn from Australia and Canada?* London: OHE, 1997.

37 Culyer A J, Posnett J. Hospital behaviour and competition. In: Culyer A J, Maynard A K, Posnett J. ed. *Competition in health care: reforming the NHS.* Basingstoke: Macmillan, 1990.

38 Robinson R. The impact of the NHS reforms 1991–1995: a review of research evidence. *J Public Health Med* 1996;**18**(3):337–42.

39 Paton C. Counting the costs. *Health Serv J* 1997;**21 August**:24–7.

40 Jost TS, Hughes D, McHale J, Griffiths L. The British health care reforms, the American health care revolution, and purchaser/provider contracts. *J Health Policy, Politics, and Law* 1995;**20**(4):887–908.

41 Propper C, Bartlett W. The impact of competition on the behaviour of National Health Service trusts. In: Flynn R, Williams G. ed. *Contracting for health: quasi-markets and the NHS.* Oxford: Oxford University Press, 1997.

42 Chalkley M Malcolmson J. Contracts for the National Health Service. *Economic J* 1996; **106**:1691–701.

43 Birch S, Gafni A. Changing the problem to fit the solution: Johanneson and Weinstein's (mis) application of economics to real world problems. *J Health Econ* 1993;**12**:469–76.

44 Briggs A, Sculpher M, Buxton MJ. Uncertainty in the economic evaluation of health care technologies: the role of sensitivity analysis. *Health Econ* 1994;**3**:95–104.

45 Sheldon TA, Maynard A. Is rationing inevitable? In: *Rationing in action.* London: BMJ Publishing Group, 1993.

46 Scott T, Wordsworth S, & Donaldson C. *Using economics in a primary care-led NHS: applying PBMA to GP fundholding.* Paper presented to HESG, Brunel, July 1996.

47 Browning M. Children and household economic behaviour. *J Econ Lit* 1992;**30**:1434–75.

48 Browning M, Deaton A, Irish M. A profitable approach to labour supply and commodity demands over the life-cycle. *Econometrica* 1985;**53**(3):503–43.

49 Mooney G. *Economics, medicine, and health care.* Hemel Hempstead: Harvester Wheatsheaf, 1992.

50 Butler JRG. *Hospital cost analysis.* London: Kluwer Academic Publishers; 1995.

51 Centre for Reviews and Dissemination. *Hospital volume and health care outcomes, costs, and patient access. Effective Health Care Bulletin 2(8).* York: NHSCRD, 1996.

52 Hamilton BH, Hamilton VH. Estimating surgical volume–outcome relationships applying survival models: accounting for frailty and hospital-fixed effects. *Health Econ* 1997;**6**(4): 383–96.

53 Langkilde LK, Sogaard J. The adjustment of cost measurement to account for learning. *Health Econ* 1997;**6**(1):83–6.

54 Birch S, Leake JL, Lewis DW. Economic issues in the development and use of practice guidelines: an application to resource allocation in dentistry. *Comm Dent Health* 1996;**13**: 70–5.

55 Walker A, Major K, Young D, Brown A. *Economic costs in the NHS: a useful insight or just bad accountancy?* Paper presented to the Health Economists' Study Group, Liverpool, 1997.

56 Torgerson DJ, Donaldson C, Garton MJ, Reid DM, Russell IT. Recruitment methods for screening programmes: the price of high compliance. *Health Econ* 1993;**2**:55–8.

57 Torgerson DJ, Gosden T. The national breast screening service: is it economically efficient? *Quart J Med* 1997;**90**:423–5.

58 Torgerson DJ, Donaldson C. An economic view of high compliance as a screening objective *BMJ* 1994;**308**:117–19.

59 Sutton M. How to get the best health outcome from a given amount of money [personal paper]. *BMJ* 1997;**315**:47–9.

60 Chapman PLH, Huygens I. An evaluation of three treatment programmes for alcoholism: an experimental study with 6- and 18-month follow-ups. *Br J Addict* 1988;**83**:67–81.

61 Torgerson D, Campbell M. Unequal randomisation can improve the economic efficiency of clinical trials. *J Health Serv Res Policy* 1997;**2**(2):81–5.

62 Whynes D K. Towards an evidence based National Health Service? *Economic J* 1996;**106**: 1702–12.

63 Escarce JJ. Externalities in hospitals and physician adoption of a new surgical technology: an exploratory analysis. *J Health Econ* 1996;**15**:715–34.

64 Hirshleifer D. The blind leading the blind. Social influence, fads, and informational cascades. In: Tomassi M, Ierulli K. ed. *The new economics of human behaviour.* Cambridge: Cambridge University Press, 1995.

65 Scott A, Hall J. Evaluating the effects of GP remuneration: problems and prospects. *Health Policy* 1995;**31**:183–95.

66 Hughes D, McGuire A. *An empirical investigation of hospital cost functions introducing output heterogeneity and controlling for demand uncertainty.* Paper presented to HESG, York, July 1997.

67 Hey J. *Experiments in economics.* Blackwell (Oxford), 1991.

68 Sheldon TA. Problems of using modelling in the economic evaluation of health care. *Health Econ* 1996;**5**:1–11.

69 Buxton MJ, Drummond MF, van Hout BA, *et al.* Modelling in economic evaluation: an unavoidable fact of life. *Health Econ* 1997;**6**;217–27.

70 McClellan M, McNeill BJ, Newhouse JP. Does more intensive treatment of acute myocardial patients in the elderly reduce mortality: analysis using instrumental variables. *JAMA* 1994;**272**:859–66.

71 Heckman JJ. Instrumental variables: a study of implicit behavioral assumptions used in making program evaluations. *J Hum Res* 1997;**XXXII**:441–61.

72 Garfinkel I, Manski CF, Michalopoulus C. Micro experiments and macro effects. In: Manski CF, Garfinkel I. ed. *Evaluating welfare and training programs.* Cambridge: Harvard University Press; 1992.

73 Philipson T, Hedges LV. Treatment evaluation through social experiments: subjects vs. investigators. Mimeo: Department of Economics, University of Chicago, 1996.

74 Weinstein MC. From cost-effectiveness ratios to resource allocation: where to draw the line? In: Sloan FA. ed. *Valuing health care: costs, benefits, and effectiveness of pharmaceuticals and other medical technologies.* Cambridge: Cambridge University Press, 1995.

15 Changing clinical practice in the light of the evidence: two contrasting stories from perinatology

VIVIENNE VAN SOMEREN

Introduction

Diffidence about incorporating new knowledge into everyday practice is widespread.[1] The nature of obstacles to desirable change has been explored and some strategies for changing clinicians' behaviour have been subjected to controlled trials.[2,3] However, the complex interactions between the nature of the intervention and the mind-set of the clinician have received less attention. Here, an analysis is offered of two interventions that produce comparable reductions in mortality from respiratory distress syndrome in preterm infants, but have very different implementation histories. The two interventions are antenatal administration of corticosteroids to the mother in threatened preterm delivery and administration of exogenous surfactant to the baby. Both reduce the risk of neonatal mortality due to respiratory distress syndrome of prematurity by 40%.[4,5]

Methods

The trial data and the history of the implementation of the interventions were reviewed in the conventional way, with computer-assisted literature searches and particular use being made of the overviews provided by the Cochrane Collaboration. Special attention was also paid to the rhetoric in editorials that accompanied new studies. The author reflected on her

143

personal experience of the introduction of surfactant and discussed her impressions of the early days of corticosteroids with more senior colleagues.

Box 15.1   Adoption of antenatal steroids for prevention of neonatal respiratory distress syndrome

1969   Liggins:[6] the physiology

1972   Liggins and Howie.[7] the first clinical trial in humans demonstrates effectiveness

1970s   Concern about untoward effects[10]

1981   American collaborative trial report[8] confirms effect, but message lost in sub-group analyses
No consensus on steroid usage in preterm labour[9]

1990   UK publication of meta-analysis confirms effects on mortality and morbidity[4]

1991   Minority of mothers of babies in Osiris (surfactant) trial receive steroids[16]

1995   Uptake still poor, so National Institutes of Health produce consensus statement[11]

Adoption of antenatal corticosteroids (Box 15.1)

In 1969, Liggins reported on the role of corticosteroids in preterm labour in sheep.[6] An unexpected finding was that steroids accelerated fetal lung maturation in the lambs. Quick to realise the potential benefits in humans, Liggins and Howie set up a controlled trial in which 282 women took part, and which was reported in 1972.[7] Although this showed a halving in perinatal mortality from 20% to 10%, the message was diluted by the presentation. For instance, the first results table shows a statistically non-significant adverse effect in a sub-group of 32 pregnancies complicated by pregnancy-induced hypertension.

A large American collaborative trial confirmed that antenatal steroids produced a great reduction in respiratory distress, but failed to find a reduction in mortality.[8] Many sub-group analyses were done and the abstract below emphasises the ensuing negative results:

> "The effect was, however, mainly attributable to discernible differences among singleton female infants (P<0.001), whereas no treatment effect was observed in male infants (P = 0.96). Non-Caucasians were improved whereas Caucasians showed little benefit. Fetal and neonatal mortality . . . were not different."[8]

Editorials of the time were cautious. There was much discussion of the sub-group analyses, emphasising that only certain categories might benefit.[9] Fears of side-effects were aired in emotive language:

"The frightening possibilities of long-term harm must be weighed against short-term benefits. Long latent periods associated with aberrant developmental expression are known in the human."[10]

The disastrous misuse of oxygen in premature babies in the 1940s and 1950s was fresh in paediatricians' minds, along with the unforeseen long-term consequences on female offspring of giving stilboestrol early in pregnancy. In addition, artificial ventilation for respiratory distress syndrome, introduced in the 1960s, had become widely available during the 1970s and produced such a dramatic fall in mortality that the steroid effect was perceived as small in comparison and not worth the risk of side-effects.

Perinatal trials were among the first to be subjected to meta-analysis. By 1990 it was finally clear that there was overwhelming evidence of benefit from the maternal administration of steroids when preterm delivery was anticipated. The odds ratio for respiratory distress syndrome is currently 0.51 (95% CI 0.42–0.61) and for neonatal death is 0.61 (95% CI 0.49–0.78).[4] However, clinicians were slow to act on this information. Surveys in the early 1990s showed that only 12–18% of eligible women were receiving treatment. Realising the magnitude of the problem in the United States, the National Institutes of Health called a consensus conference and in 1995 published unequivocal advice to obstetricians, encouraging antenatal steroids.[11]

Box 15.2 Adoption of surfactant for prevention and treatment of respiratory distress syndrome

1957   Avery and Mead:[12] the physiology
1980   First uncontrolled clinical trial[13]
1980s   Large clinical trials tend to show effectiveness[5]
1990   Osiris trial engages large numbers of neonatologists[16]
1991   UK product licence[14]
1994   Established treatment

Artificial surfactant for preterm infants (Box 15.2)

In 1959, four years after the existence of lung surfactant was first postulated, Avery and Mead demonstrated that the lungs of preterm babies dying from hyaline membrane disease were deficient in the material responsible for

145

low surface tension in adult lungs and considered the role of this deficiency in the pathogenesis of the disease.[12] The concept of respiratory distress syndrome of prematurity as a surfactant deficiency disease was adopted quickly. Thus logic demanded surfactant as treatment, but there was a long delay before chemists could produce an effective, stable compound suitable for administration to babies.

In 1980, Fujiwara *et al.* reported the first uncontrolled case series in which 10 infants with severe respiratory distress syndrome were given artificial surfactant.[13] The effects were dramatic: the change in clinical condition was so great that in three hours the babies moved out of a prognostic group in which death was highly likely into one in which survival was predicted. All survived.

The preparations that became available in the 1980s were all experimental and unlicensed and the only way surfactant could be given was as part of a controlled trial. By 1991 there had been more than 30 controlled trials, involving over 6000 babies, and meta-analysis showed that risk of death was reduced by 40% by surfactant.[5] Although potential side-effects such as antigenic sensitisation were discussed, there was less emphasis than there had been for steroids. In 1991, surfactant was licensed in Britain and there was a brief period of unjustified anxiety about whether health authorities would fund it.[14] By 1994, enough surfactant was sold in Britain to treat between 6000 and 8000 babies, enough for the 1% of UK babies likely to benefit.

Discussion

Antenatal steroids were first subjected to a controlled trial in 1972, but by 1995 there were still clinicians who doubted their value or worried about adverse effects. In contrast, artificial surfactant was subject to its first controlled trial in 1984 and uptake was virtually universal within 10 years. Why did one intervention take twice as long as the other to become normal clinical practice? The two interventions have similar impacts on the same disease. The two groups of clinicians involved, obstetricians and paediatricians, have similar scientific training and work closely together. However, there are important differences, both in the treatments themselves and in clinicians' perceptions of them (Table 15.1)

Everyday practice of obstetricians and paediatricians

For neonatal paediatricians, prematurity and respiratory distress syndrome are the cornerstones of their practice. In contrast, only 2% of antenatal patients will deliver before 32 weeks and few obstetricians spend most of

Table 13.1   Steroids and surfactant: clinicians' contrasting experiences and attitudes

	The paediatrician and surfactant	The obstetrician and steroids
Impact on everyday practice of disease	RDS is the commonest cause of death and disability in the neonatal unit	Preterm labour affects a small minority of pregnant women
Disease mechanism	RDS is a surfactant deficiency disease	Preterm labour is multifactorial and poorly understood
Prescribers' views	Effect seen in minutes. Must stand by ventilator as big changes in settings likely to be needed	Paediatricians report lowering of neonatal mortality in annual report
Conflict between two patients	No	Yes
Perception of side-effects	Dismissed too quickly	Lingering possibility of very longterm effects
Pharmaceutical interest	Yes	No
Widespread involvement in trials	Yes	No
Trial technology	Late 1980s	Early 1970s
Opinion leaders' views	For	Against

their working week with women in very preterm labour. Thus the disease is a higher priority for one group, who will naturally seek out new information related to it.

Disease mechanisms

Lung mechanics are familiar to all medical students; the physical properties of surfactant had been well established by 1960 and incorporated into the bedrock of preclinical physiology. Paediatric textbooks taught that respiratory distress of prematurity was a surfactant deficiency disease. In contrast, there is no intuitive connection between a serendipitous observation made in fetal sheep and everyday practice in the labour ward.

Immediate impact on prescriber

A paediatrician who gives a few babies surfactant is in no doubt about its effect. He or she must be prepared to alter the ventilator settings within minutes of administration. The effect is obvious and no meta-analysis is needed to convince the clinician. In contrast, an obstetrician who prescribes dexamethasone to a mother does not personally observe any effect. The effect is apparent in end-of-year perinatal mortality and morbidity meetings.

147

An obstetrician responsible for 500 births per year will experience one less death from prematurity per annum if he or she regularly prescribes steroids. One treatment produces effects appreciated by the clinician's eyes, the other by his intellect.

Side-effects and conflicts between two patients

There is widespread professional and lay concern about the side-effects of steroids. The potential adverse effects of antenatal steroids were widely discussed. For the mother there was metabolic upset, increased blood pressure, and increased susceptibility to infection. For the fetus there was all this, plus possible effects on growth and unpredictable long-term effects. Why should an obstetrician prescribe something that had definite disadvantages for one of two patients and only questionable advantages (in the light of the evidence before 1990) for the other?

In contrast, there may not have been enough concern about the side-effects of surfactants. Perhaps this was because the dominant model was of a deficiency disease. The magnitude of the early trials did mean that short-term problems, such as a 4% incidence of pulmonary haemorrhage, were quickly identified and quantified. However, the possibility of longer-term problems due to sensitisation to foreign protein still exists.

Opinion leaders and group pressure

Neonatal intensive care has a short and dazzling history. Ventilation was widely adopted in the 1970s and doubled the survival of infants under 2000g at birth.[15] The short timescale means that today's middle-aged neonatologists all sat at the feet of the small band of talented innovators who developed the specialty in the 1960s. The British neonatal community is very closeknit and once a view is held by a small number of opinion leaders it will be widely adopted. For surfactant this was a good thing, but other innovations have been introduced before full evaluation.

Obstetrics is a mature specialty with a long history. Obstetricians are more numerous than neonatologists and have more diffuse interests, usually working in both obstetrics and gynaecology. In the 1970s obstetricians embraced technological advance wholeheartedly. Following this they were subjected to criticism from their patients to a degree unparalleled in any other specialty. They are more likely to be sued than other specialists. A cautious attitude to new treatments is inevitable is such a climate of opinion.

148

Effective continuing medical education and clinician involvement in trials

Less than one in 1000 at-risk mothers treated during the 1980s were enrolled in steroid trials. In contrast, in 1990–91, about 25% of the relevant British preterm population took part in a huge trial.[16] One of the reasons for this vast difference in the exposure of the obstetric and paediatric communities to the trials was pharmaceutical company involvement. Dexamethasone, a long-established steroid preparation, costs £1.00 per treatment course. Surfactant, developed after years in the laboratory, had to be tested in the field before getting a product licence and now sells for about £300 per dose. The pharmaceutical industry was thus prepared to fund large trials.

The advantages of this were that neonatologists had early access to the material and plenty of opportunities to meet to discuss results and experiences. The magnitude of immediate side-effects was easy to assess. Collaborators' meetings were also a forum where such concepts as trial size, confidence intervals, and primary versus secondary analyses were discussed, thus providing excellent opportunities for many of us to learn about evidence based medicine.

Taking part in a well-organised clinical trial involves participants in precisely those activities which are most effective for changing clinicians' practice.[2,3] Participants are sensitised to information about the intervention from a wide variety of sources. They attend seminars which target the subject and are very interactive. They also receive reminders with every patient contact. At the end, they feel considerable ownership of the trial results.

The nature of the trial evidence

Steroid trials were begun in the 1970s. The emphasis in the reporting is on "P" values and whether the differences between groups are statistically significant. The magnitude of the effect is not emphasised. Although there are two large trials, there are also a number of small ones with conflicting results due to small numbers. Even in the large trials the message is obscured by the sub-group analyses. Thus, it was not until the data were subject to systematic review and meta-analysis that the advantages of steroids became clear. When the evidence is confusing, it is easy for highly intelligent people to find scholarly, theoretical reasons for clinging to entrenched beliefs.

Surfactant trials were carried out in the 1980s. Statistical techniques had become more sophisticated. The importance of adequate sample size, reporting on an intention-to-treat basis, reporting the size of observed

149

effects with confidence intervals, and avoiding *post hoc* sub-group analyses were all appreciated. Thus, surfactant trials are easier to read individually than steroid trials and meta-analyses are easier to conduct.

With hindsight, the clinicians who were cautious about antenatal steroids were wrong. Some of the non-scientific reasons are explored above. However, in the 1980's, there remained real scientific uncertainty. What was the meaning of the subgroup analyses? How bad might steroid side effects be in women with hypertension? What about infection if the membranes were ruptured? Were the trial results still valid in an era of improving neonatal intensive care and falling death rates? Today, with the technology of evidence based medicine more clearly appreciated, some of these questions could be resolved more quickly. However, the clinician faced with trial evidence will always have to make judgements about whether the trial circumstances match the individual patient's circumstances closely enough that the trial results are relevant *today* for *this* patient.

Conclusions

Neither the nature of the intervention nor its scientific pedigree can fully explain why one innovation is adopted quickly and another slowly. This analysis has shown the importance of clinicians' previous assumptions and beliefs and the cultural framework in which they work. The conclusion accords both with common sense and with academic exploration of adult learning and behaviour.[17,18]

However, the literature of continuing medical education has emphasised the cognitive aspects of learning at the expense of the social, personal, environmental, and behavioural factors to which we are all subject. Clinicians seeking to practise and teach evidence based medicine must learn to look for the seemingly irrational in themselves as well as in their colleagues. We should consider our previous experience and preconceptions in order to remove the barriers to new ideas.

References

1 Noble J. Influence of physician perceptions in putting knowledge into practice. *Lancet* 1996;**347**:1571.
2 Wensing M, Grol R. Single and combined strategies for implementing changes in primary care: a literature review. *Int J Qual Health Care* 1994;**6**:115–32.
3 Davis DA, Thomson MA. Oxman AD, Haynes B. Changing physician performance: a systematic review of the effect of continuing medical education strategies. *JAMA* 1995; **274**:700–5.
4 Crowley P. Corticosteroids prior to preterm delivery. In: Enkin MW, Keirse MJNC, Renfrew MJ, Neilson JP. ed. *Pregnancy and Childbirth Module*. Cochrane Database of Systematic Reviews: Review No 02955, 5 May 1994.

5 Soll F, McQueen MC. Respiratory distress syndrome. in: Sinclair JC, Bracken MB. ed. *Effective care of the newborn infant.* Oxford: Oxford University Press, 1992.

6 Liggins GC. Premature delivery of foetal lambs infused with glucocorticoids. *J Endocr* 1969;**45**:515.

7 Liggins GC, Howie RN. A controlled trial of antepartum glucocorticoid treatment for prevention of the respiratory distress syndrome in premature infants. *Pediatrics* 1972;**50**: 515–25.

8 Collaborative group on antenatal steroid therapy. Effect of antenatal dexamethasone administration on the prevention of respiratory distress syndrome. *Am J Obstet. Gynecol* 1981;**141**:276–87.

9 Little B. Editorial comment. *Am J Obs Gyn* 1981;**141**:287.

10 Gluck L. Administration of corticosteroids to induce maturation of fetal lung. *Am J Dis Child* 1976;**130**:976–8.

11 NIH Consensus Conference. Effect of corticosteroids for fetal maturation on perinatal outcomes. *JAMA* 1995;**273**:413–18.

12 Avery ME, Mead J. Surface properties in relation to atelectasis and hyaline membrane disease. *Am J Dis Child* 1959;**97**:517–23.

13 Fujiwara T, Maeta H, Chida S, *et al.* Artificial surfactant therapy in hyaline-membrane disease. *Lancet* 1980;**1**:55–9.

14 Halliday H. Introducing new cost-effective treatments into the NHS. Surfactant treatment for premature babies: who cares enough to pay? *Qual Health Care* 1993;**2**:195–7.

15 Cooke RI, Davis PA. The care of newborn babies – some developments and dilemnas. In: Forfar JO. ed. Child health in a changing society. Oxford: Oxford University Press, 1988.

16 The Osiris Collaborative Group. Early versus delayed neonatal administration of synthetic surfactant – the judgement of OSIRIS. *Lancet* p 1363–69.

17 Nowlem PM. *A new approach to continuing education for business and the professions.* New York, NY: Macmillan, 1988.

18 Bandura A. *Social foundations of thought and action: a social cognitive theory.* Englewood Cliffs, NJ: Prentice Hall, 1986.

Index

153